Materials and Procedures
for Today's Dental Assistant

Materials and Procedures
for Today's Dental Assistant

Ellen Dietz-Bourguignon

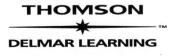
THOMSON

DELMAR LEARNING

Australia   Canada   Mexico   Singapore   Spain   United Kingdom   United States

THOMSON
™
DELMAR LEARNING

Materials and Procedures for Today's Dental Assistant
by Ellen Dietz-Bourguignon

Vice President,
Health Care Business Unit:
William Brottmiller

Editorial Director:
Cathy L. Esperti

Acquisitions Editor:
Maureen Rosener

Developmental Editor:
Laurie Traver

Marketing Director:
Jennifer McAvey

Marketing Coordinator:
Christopher Manion

Editorial Assistant:
Elizabeth Howe

Technology Project Manager:
Mary Colleen Liburdi

Production Editor:
Bridget Lulay

Library of Congress Cataloging-in-Publication Data

Dietz-Bourguignon, Ellen.
  Materials and procedures for today's dental assistant / Ellen Dietz-Bourguignon.
   p. ; cm.
  Includes bibliographical references and index.
  ISBN 1-4018-3733-6 (pbk.)
  1. Dental materials.   2. Dental assistants.
  [DNLM: 1. Dental Materials.   2. Dental Assistants.   WU 190 D566m 2005] I. Title.
  RK652.5.D54 2005
  617.690233—dc22

                              2004029709

Notice to the Reader

Publisher does not warrant or guarantee any of the products described herein or perform any independent analysis in connection with any of the product information contained herein. Publisher does not assume, and expressly disclaims, any obligation to obtain and include information other than that provided to it by the manufacturer.

The reader is expressly warned to consider and adopt all safety precautions that might be indicated by the activities described herein and to avoid all potential hazards. By following the instructions contained herein, the reader willingly assumes all risks in connection with such instructions.

The publisher makes no representations or warranties of any kind, including but not limited to, the warranties of fitness for particular purpose or merchantability, nor any such representations implied with respect to the material set forth herein, and the publisher takes no responsibility with respect to such material. The publisher shall not be liable for any special, consequential, or exemplary damages resulting, in whole or part, from the reader's use of, or reliance upon, this material.

This book is dedicated to M_____ always in my heart. And to m_____ husband, partner, and best friend _____ love is the light of my life. Thank _____ teaching me patienc_____rt . . . and that home is wh_____ we are together.

CONTENTS

Section I   Cements and Liners   23

Chapter 2   Preliminary Restorative Dental Materials   25

Section IV   Gypsum Materials   145

Chapter 6   Dental Gypsum Materials   147

Section V   Related Dental Materials   167

Chapter 7   Dental Waxes   169

Chapter 10   **Miscellaneous Dental Materials and Hazardous Substances**   **230**

Appendix A   **Dental Assisting National Board, Inc. Task Analysis, General Chairside Tasks**   **251**

Appendix B   **Textbook Figures Found on Accompanying StudyWARE™ CD-ROM**   **253**

It is exciting when a new product like *Materials and Procedures for Today's Dental Assistant* addresses the needs of the busy dental practitioner and educator. Teaching hands-on skills is a tedious and sometimes frustrating task since each component of the procedure must be broken down for the new learner and each learner progresses at a different pace. Experienced clinicians and educators often have difficulty processing information at this very basic level, so they often have difficulty in teaching at the novice level. This text breaks the tasks down into easy, understandable components that are objective and measurable. This book is ideally suited to provide students with the step-by-step instructions needed to master new procedures while allowing the learner to progress at his or her own pace.

Educational research tells us that the adult learner must repeat tasks or learning concepts six to eight times before they are committed to memory, and the concept of the Practice Makes Perfect sheets reinforces this concept. Dental materials have always presented a challenge to the instructor because precision is necessary for successful manipulation, but time and personnel constraints are always present. The Practice Makes Perfect worksheets give specific criteria that must be met for achieving competence and provide the feedback and guidance that both the learner and the educator need.

Today's learner needs the visual format, and the images provided in the book and CD-ROM allow students to compare their efforts to the product desired and to reinforce the visual-neural learning pathway. The additional quiz questions and sequencing activities help develop the theoretical background needed to process new information. As dental materials continue to change and evolve, this type of text is especially helpful since it focuses on critical tasks and information. As the learner masters each procedure, he or she will gain the confidence needed to be a competent dental assistant. This text is destined to be a valuable resource in the rewarding process of guiding tomorrow's dental professionals.

Dr. Bob Bennett, BS, DMD
Department Co-Chair,
Dental Assisting and
Dental Hygiene Programs
Texas State Technical College
Harlingen, TX

The role of the professional dental assistant is an ever-evolving one. Continuous changes and upgrades in the quality and ease of use of dental products and materials mandate the timely release of information and training materials for members of the dental team. Whether a student, an on-the-job trained assistant, or a dental assistant searching out a review text prior to taking the national certification examination, *Materials and Procedures for Today's Dental Assistant* is intended to be a useful educational tool.

■ Intended Audience and Use

Materials and Procedures for Today's Dental Assistant reflects the latest in dental materials in a reader- and student-friendly format. It guides the dental assisting student through relevant information and exercises to use in a clinical dental setting and in the dental office laboratory. This book may also be helpful as a refresher for dental assistants employed in private practice and for those seeking a review text to prepare for the national Infection Control Exam administered by the Dental Assisting National Board (DANB). It is recommended that the user have basic knowledge of and familiarity with dental terminology, dental anatomy, dental instrumentation, and the role of the dental assistant.

In keeping with national standards required for certification of dental assistants, *Materials and Procedures for Today's Dental Assistant* addresses all requirements set forth by the DANB Task Analysis, Chicago, Illinois, to prepare for the national certification examination at the time of publication. Candidates for the DANB Certification Examination are encouraged to contact DANB periodically to inquire about updates or changes in the requirements.

Completion of the content herein, including but not limited to the chapter material, Practice Makes Perfect Student Assessment Sheets, and StudyWARE CD-ROM, does not imply a guarantee of successful completion or a passing score on the DANB Certification Examination.

■ Organization and Features

For ease of instruction and learning, *Materials and Procedures for Today's Dental Assistant* is divided into the following five sections, according to their relevance to the dental assistant's role in chairside assisting, laboratory work, and related information:

  I. Cements and Liners
 II. Restorative Materials
III. Impression Materials
 IV. Gypsum Materials
  V. Related Dental Materials

Within these five sections, there are several pedagogical features that help to make this book reader and student friendly, which will enhance the learning experience. Following is a summary of these features:

Learning Objectives, Key Terms, and Glossary

Learning Objectives and Key Terms appear at the beginning of each chapter. Learning objectives provide students a preview of what they can expect to learn in the chapter, and key terms, which are boldfaced in their first appearance in the chapter, help to reinforce specific terms with which the student should be familiar. These terms are also defined in the Glossary, which is located at the back of the text.

Critical Thinking and Posttest Questions

Critical Thinking Questions are found near the end of each chapter, preceding Practice Makes Perfect Student Assessments and Posttest Questions. Not only do critical thinking questions help students assess their comprehension and retention of the material, but they also encourage critical thinking skills, which are crucial for dental assistants and other health care professionals to demonstrate in the workplace.

Posttest Questions can be found at the end of each chapter of the book. The posttest questions, like the critical thinking questions, allow students to assess their retention and comprehension of the material they have read in the chapter and help students know on which areas they might need to spend more time. These questions are multiple choice, and several of them are written in a format that poses the question using the word *except* in italics, which further encourages critical thinking because students must think on more than one level to reach the correct answer.

Practice Makes Perfect (PMP) Procedures and Student Assessments

Numerous hands-on procedures are outlined in Practice Makes Perfect Procedures, also referred to as PMP procedures, and are designed to help the reader put into practice the information and techniques outlined and learned in Chapters 2 through 9. Students and instructors should be aware that the armamentarium listed at the beginning of each Practice Makes Perfect Procedure include only the *minimum* of equipment and instruments required for the classroom or laboratory setting. In an actual dental office or laboratory environment, additional hand and rotary instruments and other related accessories will be necessary. To help the reader visualize certain steps in procedures, photos or diagrams are included in some PMP procedures. Also note that in some PMP procedures the reader will be directed to a previous section or to another chapter for additional information or instructions.

Practice Makes Perfect Student Assessments are also included at the end of Chapters 2 through 9. The procedures covered in the Student Assessments correspond to the PMP procedures but are intended more for the instructor to assess the student's mastery of skills in working with specific dental materials covered in the chapter. The instructional tips that are included in the procedure sheets are omitted from the assessment sheets, and instructors are provided space at the end of the assessments to make notes on how the student completed the procedure. Students may cut the PMP procedure and assessment sheets out of the book or they can print the sheets from the StudyWARE CD-ROM.

StudyWARE™ CD-ROM

The StudyWARE CD-ROM is a student activity disk that is included with the book. The disk is intended to enhance the student's learning of the material covered in the chapters by providing a variety of activities and question types. Quiz questions are interactive, with automatic feedback provided for correct and incorrect answers. Providing this type of feedback results in quizzes that are learning activities for the students as well as assessments of knowledge and comprehension.

Students can also test their knowledge of procedures with sequencing exercises, which require the student to put steps of selected procedures from the book into the correct order. Case studies with accompanying questions are another activity which encourage critical thinking. A championship game that combines the quiz questions into one game is a fun way for students, either on their own or in a classroom setting, to test the knowledge they have gained from all chapters in the book. Selected figures from the book have also been provided on the StudyWARE. The figures provided on the StudyWARE are in color, which will enable students to more effectively see certain characteristics of materials such as consistency and differences in color. A list of these figures can be found in Appendix B (page 253) of this book.

PPE Icons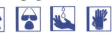

Specific icons are provided to depict additional necessary items required to ensure protection against bloodborne disease transmission, including handwashing, gloves, masks, eyewear, and personal protective equipment (PPE). These icons are included at the beginning of each PMP procedure to remind students of the importance of always using the appropriate PPE.

Charts and Forms

To facilitate learning and putting into practice the concepts introduced throughout this text, many useful charts and forms have been included. These may be reproduced by the instructor or student for classroom practice and laboratory exercises.

■ Thank You

Many wonderful people have contributed their time and talents in making *Materials and Procedures for Today's Dental Assistant* possible. Heartfelt thanks deservedly go to Katherine Green of Tempe, Arizona, and to Virginia S. Helms, CDA, EFDA, of Albuquerque, New Mexico, for their support, encouragement, and many hours of proofreading; also to employees and friends of Banner Health Arizona, who periodically asked, "How's the book coming?"

Thanks are also extended to the dedicated staff of Thomson Delmar Learning, including editors, administrative support people, sales and marketing representatives, and graphic designers.

And finally, thanks are due to the academic reviewers who have given of their experience and wisdom in reviewing chapters and providing valuable feedback. Their names are provided following the preface.

■ Concluding Thoughts

We wish you every success in your pursuit of learning more about dental materials using *Materials and Procedures for Today's Dental Assistant,* and we welcome feedback from instructors and students on their experiences in using this text.

ACKNOWLEDGMENTS

Dr. Bob Bennett, BS, DMD
Department Co-Chair
Dental Assisting and Dental Hygiene
  Programs
Texas State Technical College
Harlingen, TX

Susan Walmer Burton, DMD, DH, DA
Dental Director of Eastern State Hospital
Director of Dr. Burton's Dental Auxiliary
  Course
Private Practice
Lexington, KY

Christina Discello, CDA, AST
Instructor, Dental Assisting
Coordinator of Community Services
Career Training Academy
New Kensington, PA

Patricia A Frese, RDH, MEd
Professor in Dental Hygiene
University of Cincinnati, Raymond Walters
  College
Cincinnati, OH

Terri Heintz, CDA, RDA
Dental Assisting Instructor
Health and Public Services Department
Des Moines Area Community College
Des Moines, IA

Stella Lovato, CDA, MSHP, MA
Professor and Program Coordinator
Dental Assisting Chair
Allied Health
San Antonio College/ACCD
San Antonio, TX

Barbara Stackhouse, RDH, MEd
Dental Hygienist/Practice Development
  Coach
Schuster Center for Professional
  Development
Scottsdale, AZ

Kris Tupper BS, CDA, EFDA, EFODA
Dental Assisting Instructor
Lane Community College
Eugene, OR

Lynn Marie Wilson, CDA, EFDA, MS.Ed.
Health Academy Director/Health
  Occupations Educator
Portage Township School Corporation
Portage, IN

*A special thank-you is extended to Stella Lovato
for her insightful contributions to the final
manuscript and to Barbara Stackhouse for her
conscientious and diligent efforts on the
StudyWARE CD-ROM.*

Ellen Dietz-Bourguignon has enjoyed a successful 35-year dental career, beginning as an associate-degreed CDA (a graduate of Dutchess Community College, Poughkeepsie, NY) and in private practice. After working as a chairside assistant and office manager, she returned to college and earned her Bachelor of Science Degree in Allied Health Education in Dental Auxiliary Utilization and a Community College Teaching Certificate from the State University of New York at Buffalo.

Following a combined seven-year dental assisting teaching career at Orange County Community College, the University of North Carolina at Chapel Hill, Erie County BOCES, and Niagara County Community College, she began to pursue her true love, writing about dentistry.

Ellen initially accepted the Front Desk Column of *Dental Assisting Magazine* and one year later took over the managing editor post. In the following years, she worked in dental marketing, project management, and product development at Semantodontics (SmartPractice/SmartHealth) and as editor of *PracticeSmart Newsletter;* she also worked in legal administration for the Arizona State Board of Dental Examiners.

Ellen has published ten books in the dental assisting field, including *Delmar's Dental Office Management, Delmar's Dental Assisting Curriculum Guide, Lesson Plans for the Dental Assistant, Safety Standards and Infection Control for Dental Assistants,* and *Safety Standards and Infection Control for Dental Hygienists,* and was a contributing author to *The Dental Assistant.* She is a member of OSAP and has been a speaker and keynote speaker at ADAA Annual Sessions.

Ellen has authored numerous accredited continuing dental education home study programs and is editor of *The Explorer,* published by the National Association of Dental Assistants, of Falls Church, Virginia. Her articles have appeared in *JADAA: The Dental Assistant, Dental Assisting, DENTIST, The Dental Student, Dental Economics, RDH, CONTACT,* and *Dental Teamwork Magazine.*

Ellen is also founder and executive director of Toothbrushes for Tomorrow™, a nonprofit organization dedicated to the principle that no child should be without a toothbrush.

PRACTICE MAKES PERFECT PROCEDURES

Following is a list of the PMP (Practice Makes Perfect) procedures found in this book. Each PMP procedure has a corresponding Student Assessment sheet, which can be found at the end of the chapter (Chapters 2 through 9). The Student Assessment sheets are also available on the accompanying StudyWARE CD-ROM, so students may print the assessments out if they prefer, rather than cutting them out of the book.

INTRODUCTION TO DENTAL MATERIALS AND THE DENTAL ENVIRONMENT

LEARNING OBJECTIVES

Upon completion of this chapter the student should be able to:

1. List the general uses and categories of dental materials.

2. List and describe the 18 properties of dental materials outlined, including considerations for their use in dentistry.

3. Describe the use, necessity, rationale, and components of universal (standard) precautions and personal protective equipment (PPE) when performing invasive dental procedures or working with dental materials and when performing related dental laboratory procedures.

4. Relate the importance of communication with the commercial dental laboratory, maintaining a case tracking system, and handling of impressions, prostheses, and appliances before and after patient treatment.

5. Describe the role of the dental assistant or office manager relevant to dental supply and materials ordering, inventory control, and shelf life.

KEY TERMS

acidity	malleability
adhesion	microleakage
alkalinity	personal protective
armamentarium	equipment (PPE)
biting forces	retention
corrosion	shelf life
dimensional change	solubility
ductility	thermal properties
elasticity	toxicity (toxic effects)
esthetics	universal (standard)
flow	precautions
galvanism	viscosity
hardness	wettability

■ INTRODUCTION

The role of the dental assistant in working with dental materials is a significant one. As such, this introductory chapter is divided into three parts: general uses and categories of dental materials; the importance of following universal (standard) precautions, sound infection control, and asepsis in the dental office laboratory; and dental supply ordering and inventory control.

It is important that the dental assistant have an overall introduction and review of these concepts prior to working with dental materials, whether assisting the dentist at chairside or working in the dental office laboratory.

■ GENERAL USES AND CATEGORIES OF DENTAL MATERIALS

Many dental supplies and products are used in the dental office on a daily basis. Dental materials are categorized according to their functions or uses in the oral cavity.

Chairside dental materials include liners, cavity varnishes, and dental cements and bases; composite and amalgam restorations; primary and secondary impression materials; waxes and acrylics; and anticariogenics, surgical packings, dressings, and bleaches. Laboratory dental materials include gypsum and resin products. Other materials used in dentistry include radiographic chemistry and dental disinfectants.

Dental materials and supplies are regulated and tested for product claims and safety before becoming available for use. The American Dental Association (ADA) and the Food and Drug Administration (FDA) regulate dental materials and devices. The ADA Council on Dental Materials, Instruments, and Equipment is responsible for the information dissemination and testing of dental materials; it periodically publishes a list of certified dental materials in the *Journal of the American Dental Association (JADA)* and in *Clinical Products in Dentistry: A Desktop Reference.*

The ADA Seal of Certification denotes that the dental material or product has met the criteria established by the ADA and the U.S. government and is deemed safe and effective. The ADA Council also administers the Seal of Acceptance, which indicates that a new material has been proven safe and effective through biological, laboratory, and clinical evaluation; however, there are no physical standards of specification by which the material can be measured for certification.

■ ORAL ENVIRONMENT AND DENTAL MATERIALS

The oral cavity provides a unique environment mainly because of its harsh conditions and their effects upon dental materials. Materials must be as inert and biocompatible with the oral environment as possible as well as be durable and cost-effective.

The oral cavity environment is moist and is subject to fluctuations in acidity, significant grinding and stress factors, and rapid temperature changes. These factors require that guidelines be set forth for the development of compatible dental materials. Ideal characteristics of dental materials are listed in order of importance in Table 1-1.

General Characteristics	Specific Examples
Biocompatibility	Nontoxic, nonirritating, nonallergenic
Stability/durability	Mechanically strong, fracture resistant, hard/stiff
Resistance to corrosion and chemical effects	Durable over time
Dimensional stability	Minimally affected by solvents or temperature changes
Minimal conductivity (thermally and electrically)	Insulators
Esthetics	Closely match/replicate oral tissue appearance
Ease of manipulation	Placement and finishing with reasonable time and effort for the operator
Adherence to oral tissues	Provides durable, tight adhesion/bonding for retention and sealing
Free from taste/odors	Nonirritating, nonstinging, pleasant-tasting
Ease of cleanliness/maintenance	Easy to maintain, easy to repair, easy to keep clean
Cost-effectiveness	Must be affordable to the patient

Table 1-1 Characteristics of the Ideal Dental Material

■ ROLE OF THE DENTAL ASSISTANT

The role of the dental assistant in the use of dental materials, whether at chairside or in the laboratory setting, is a significant one. The dental assistant must be familiar with the tray set-ups and **armamentarium** (equipment and supplies) required as well as with the composition, mixing and manipulation techniques, and clean-up procedures.

Some states allow the trained dental assistant to perform expanded duties, including chairside duties involving the placement of some dental materials into the oral cavity (Figure 1-1).

The dental assistant should check with the respective Board of Dental Examiners in the state of employment or the Dental Assisting National Board's website to request a list of specific allowable duties. In general, most duties allowed to be performed by the dental assistant are referred to as reversible; that is, they are temporary procedures performed under

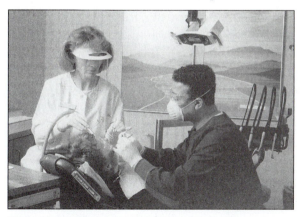

Figure 1-1 The trained dental assistant works with the dentist at chairside, using a wide varity of dental materials.

the direct supervision of the dentist or are part of an irreversible duty performed by the dentist.

■ PROPERTIES OF DENTAL MATERIALS

Dental materials are used to replace the natural dentition or portions of it, to preserve existing dentition, or to strengthen or enhance the existing esthetic appearance. The oral cavity presents a unique and complex set of environmental characteristics; thus, materials created to withstand the conditions found in the oral cavity must be developed with consideration of some of these unique factors. These factors include the following.

Acidity

The pH level of the human mouth can vary significantly. The normal pH level is approximately neutral at pH 7. (Numbers on the pH scale below 7 indicate **acidity**; numbers above 7 measure **alkalinity**.)

Humans ingest foods that may be acidic, such as citrus or tomatoes. Some of the bacteria normally growing in dental plaque are also acidic. Nonmetallic materials used in the oral cavity tend to deteriorate when constantly exposed to an overly acidic or alkaline environment. Metallic restorations may discolor or corrode when the pH at their surface is altered.

The saliva plays a role in the reduction of oral acidity. However, dental materials are subject to varying amounts of acid tolerance. How these materials react to changing acidity levels in the oral cavity determines their suitability for use in the mouth.

Another consideration with regard to suitability of use of dental materials is their potential to cause irritation to the oral tissues, specifically the gingiva and related soft tissues (oral mucosa). For example, members of the chairside dental team must take great care when using materials such as phosphoric acid (used in etching enamel and dentin), which could burn soft tissues, or to protect the eyes when using certain manufacturers' dental lights or lasers to polymerize resin-based materials.

Adhesion

In dentistry, **adhesion** is defined as the force or attraction that holds unlike substances together through physical or chemical means. Chemical adhesion is strong and more desirable with regard to dental materials; however, physical adhesion is more common.

In dentistry the adhesion process is a means to attach solid structures together. An example of chemical adhesion is the use of dental cements for luting fixed crowns and bridges; an example of physical adhesion is dental plaque and bacteria attaching as a film to the enamel.

Biting Forces

Dental materials must be of sufficient strength to withstand the **biting forces** of the human jaws. Biting force has been computed at 25,000 pounds per square inch (psi) on a single tooth in the human dentition! Molars exhibit the greatest biting force because they have the largest surface area and total cubic measurement and perform grinding motions.

The nature of human dentition is that natural teeth can withstand significantly greater biting force than prosthetic replacements, such as full and partial dentures and bridges.

Force is any push or pull on an object; the result is resistance. The reaction of the object to resist the external force is stress. When too much stress is placed on an object, this object is forced to change; this change is known as strain.

To further break this down, there are three types of stress and strain: tensile, compressive, and shearing.

Tensile Stress

Tensile stress and strain pull and stretch a material; the structure tends to become elongated. An example of tensile stress and strain is elastic rubber bands used in orthodontic treatment. The ability of a material to withstand forces of tensile stress without failing or becoming altered is called ductility.

Compressive Stress

Compressive stress and strain push or compress the material together; an example is chewing or biting. The ability of a dental material to withstand compressive stresses and strains without fracturing is called malleability.

Shearing Stress

Shearing stress and strain occur when one part of the material slides parallel to another, usually in a back-and-forth motion. An example of this in dentistry is bruxism, which is a gnashing or grinding of the teeth, often when the patient is asleep and unaware of the habit.

Color and Esthetics

Physical appearance and vanity play an increasing role in patients' acceptance of dental restorations. With regard to dental restorative materials, **esthetics** means a pleasant or attractive appearance, one that matches or enhances the patient's original (natural) dentition.

The color system of tooth shade matching is based upon three indices: hue, value, and chroma. Hue refers to the dominant color of an object: red, yellow, or blue. Value refers to the lightness of a color, on a scale from 1 to 10, with 1 meaning black and 10 meaning white. Natural teeth are generally high in value, in the range of 5–8 for most patients. Chroma is the intensity of the color on a scale from 1 to 10, in which 10 means saturated. More specifically, is the object rich in color or somewhat pale? Natural teeth are relatively low in chroma, in the range of 1–3.

Translucency

Translucency refers to the amount of light entering the tooth. Some of the light may be transmitted completely through the object or part of it may be reflected from its surface and not penetrate the tooth. Yet another part of the light may enter the object and be scattered and subsequently absorbed. If a tooth were completely clear, it would be transparent (as a pane of window glass) and there would be no light absorption. Conversely, if the tooth did not transmit any light, it would be opaque and would totally absorb the light.

Tooth edges are more transparent than the bulk of the natural tooth because the enamel is more transparent than the inner layer of dentin; edges actually appear more bluish than the thicker portion of the tooth. Light passing through the middle portion of the tooth is influenced by both enamel and dentin, and because dentin is more opaque, less light passes through this portion of the tooth; in turn, the tooth does not appear very translucent.

If a natural tooth were replaced by an artificial one that was of a uniform translucency, it would appear unnatural. The gingival portion of the tooth is usually more reddish than the rest of the tooth. This is because the reddishness of the gums is mirrored by the tooth at the gumline.

Dental ceramic and composite materials are manufactured with varying degrees of translucency for use in specific portions of a tooth. Opaquing agents (often metal oxide particles such as titanium oxide) are added to block light penetration. These materials are often used to cover up a material structure and to make the artificial tooth appear white instead of metallic. Different colors of ceramics or composites are then added to the opaque layer to make the restoration appear more natural.

Corrosion

Corrosion occurs as the result of chemical or electrochemical influences of the oral environment on metals, such as amalgam or gold. Sometimes components of food and saliva react with metals and eventually cause deep pitting or roughness. Sometimes metals in the oral cavity become dull or discolored; this effect is called tarnish (Figure 1-2).

Dimensional Change

Dimensional change in dental materials is a change in length or volume of a material, and it occurs for a variety of reasons, including the

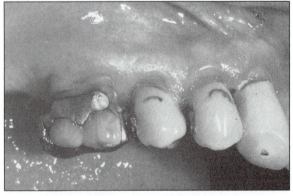

Figure 1-2 Amalgam restoration with corrosion and tarnish.

(Courtesy of Dr. Gary Shellerud.)

setting process, exposure to heat or cold associated with storage prior to activation, or exposure to foods or drink introduced into the oral cavity.

The dimensional change that occurs in dental materials is often measured by percentage of the original volume or length. Impression materials may undergo change by taking on or losing liquid. The process by which a dental material takes on additional liquid is called imbibition; the resulting stiffness is called turgor.

Dimensional change is cause for concern when selecting specific dental impression or restorative materials because the final prosthesis or restoration may not satisfactorily fit the tooth or the oral cavity.

Ductility and Malleability

The ability of a material to withstand permanent deformity under tensile stress without fracturing is known as **ductility**. If the metal is being compressed, its ability to withstand permanent deformity under compressive stress without rupturing is called **malleability**. (Ductility and malleability are usually associated with metals or wires used by the dentist.)

For example, if a metal or a dental alloy can be readily pulled into a wire, it is said to be ductile; if the metal can be hammered or rolled into a thin sheet, it is malleable. In dentistry, gold is the most ductile and malleable metal restorative. Many metals used in dentistry are both malleable and ductile.

Both malleability and ductility are reflective of the ability of a metal to be bent, contoured, or permanently deformed without fracturing. A ductile substance usually is strong; however, strength is not a required property for malleability.

Elasticity

Elasticity is the ability of a material to be distorted or deformed by applied force or the addition of a catalyst to that material; the material then returns to its original shape when the force has been removed. A common example is that of a rubber band, which, once stretched and then released, returns to its original size.

If, however, the rubber band is stretched too far or for too long, it eventually reaches its elastic limit, meaning it no longer has the ability to return to its original shape or length.

Elastic modulus is the measure of the stillness of a dental material below the elastic limit; it measures how a material can resist change or deformation.

Flow

Flow, sometimes referred to as creep, is a continuing deformation of a solid when it is under constant force. For example, some dental waxes and dental impression materials exhibit flow; dental amalgam is also subject to flow when it is placed under constant compressive forces.

Galvanism

Galvanism occurs when two different metals are present in the oral cavity and there exists a potential for a minute electrical shock. Saliva acts as the conductor of the shock between the two metals, similar to the way water conducts a shock from one entity to another during a thunder and lightning storm or when an electrical shock is created by a battery.

In dentistry, a galvanic shock may occur in the mouth of a patient who has both amalgam (silver alloy) and gold restorations.

Hardness

Hardness is the ability of a dental material to withstand or resist scratching or indentation. Dental materials lacking hardness that can be scratched or dented may eventually demonstrate wear patterns in the mouth. These are sometimes referred to as wear facets. Hardness may also cause wearing away of natural teeth as a result of frequent contact with dental materials that are harder than enamel.

Microleakage

A microscopic space always exists between a restoration and the tooth. Fluids, microorganisms, and debris from the mouth can penetrate the outer margins of the restoration and go down the walls of the cavity preparation. Eventually, this will lead to a phenomenon called **microleakage** (Figure 1-3).

Microleakage due to recurrent caries and dental sensitivity is the primary reason dental restorations must be removed and replaced. Further, the accumulation of debris in the area between the margin and the restoration increases the potential for tooth staining or discoloration. Sometimes, microleakage may cause the tooth to be sensitive to temperature

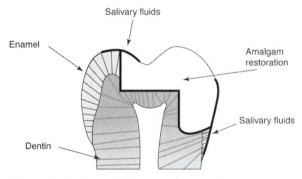

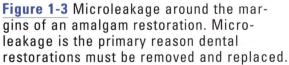

Figure 1-3 Microleakage around the margins of an amalgam restoration. Microleakage is the primary reason dental restorations must be removed and replaced.

changes following placement of a restoration. If the microleakage is severe, the pulp is continually irritated by the fluids, microorganisms, and debris that penetrate around the restoration, through the dentin, and eventually into the pulp. This can lead to an inflammatory reaction that results in pain and eventual pulp necrosis (death). Amalgam and composite restorations may be subject to microleakage.

Dental varnish is an example of a material designed to help seal out marginal caries (see *Chapter 2: Preliminary Restorative Dental Materials*).

Retention

Retention is the process by which certain materials attach to hard and soft tissues in the mouth. There are two types of retention relevant to dentistry: mechanical and chemical.

Using mechanical retention, the dentist makes specific (retentive) grooves or undercuts using a high- or low-speed handpiece in the walls of the cavity preparation or at the margins of a crown preparation to help the final restoration fit.

Chemical retention requires a chemical reaction between the tooth surface and the dental material.

Resins, cements, and bonding agents are retained on the tooth surface by either mechanical or chemical retention.

Solubility

Solubility is the ability of a substance to dissolve in a fluid. In dentistry, the solubility of a dental material is a significant factor used to determine the long-term success of the material used in the mouth.

Soluble materials may be used as bases or liners, where they are not exposed directly to saliva or liquids ingested by the patient. They are not used as final restorative materials.

Thermal Properties

Two significant **thermal properties** relevant to dental materials are thermal conductivity and thermal expansion. Thermal conductivity is the characteristic that determines the rate at which heat flows through a material. Heat capacity is the amount of heat required to raise the temperature of an object by a certain amount. This is a consideration when working with materials that are placed near the dental pulp or the gingiva.

Temperatures of the oral cavity can fluctuate significantly; the range can be as great as 150°F with the introduction of hot and cold liquids and foods. Thermal expansion occurs when the dental material is subjected to heat: It expands, then shrinks when the heat source is removed.

Temperature variations may cause dental restorative materials to expand, to shrink, to crack, or to produce undesirable dimensional changes.

Thus, the dentist must consider the thermal properties of specific materials when using them as liners and impression materials, for final restorations, or when making prostheses. Ideally, dental materials should have approximately the same thermal properties as those of natural dental structures.

Toxicity (Toxic Effects)

Few if any dental materials are completely inert. Thus, an important biological consideration is the effect the dental materials have on living tissues. Dental materials should be free of having a harmful effect on living tissues. The degree to which the material is harmful is referred to as **toxicity**. If the material is harmful, it will have a **toxic effect**.

Some dental cements, for example, require the use of a phosphoric acid liquid. Use of acidic materials could result in irritation to the pulp unless proper care is used to protect the tooth. Undesirable effects on the pulp also may be produced by chemical reactions that happen during the setting or hardening of certain restorative materials after they are placed in the oral cavity.

In its pure form in nature, fluoride, recognized for many years as an effective caries preventive substance, is poisonous. Mercury, used to make amalgam restorations, can also be toxic to humans and animals in very high doses. It is important to note, however, that when used correctly, in the recommended amounts, these two materials should pose no harm to human health.

Dental materials should be as nonirritating to the tissues as possible. They should not produce allergic or sensitizing effects on the underlying tissues.

Viscosity

Viscosity is the ability of a liquid to flow; the more viscous the substance, the stickier the substance, the less likely it is to flow quickly. Molasses is an example of a viscous substance. When heated, molasses is less viscous; when cooled, it is more viscous.

Wettability

Wettability is the ability of a material to flow over a hard or solid surface. This is significant when applying certain dental materials to the oral cavity. Wettability can be demonstrated by watching the shape of a drop on a solid material (Figure 1-4). If the drop spreads out (forming a low contact angle), the solid is quickly wetted by the material. If, however, the drop beads up (forming

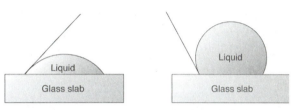

Figure 1-4 Comparison of wettability of two dental materials. The drop on the left has high wettability; the drop on the right has low wettability.

a high contact angle), the solution has poor wetting of the solid.

■ UNIVERSAL (STANDARD) PRECAUTIONS AND PERSONAL PROTECTIVE EQUIPMENT

To be protected from bloodborne diseases and other hazards associated with employment in the dental office, all members of the dental team who as a routine part of their job may encounter exposure to body fluids such as blood or saliva (Category I and Category II workers) must employ **universal (standard) precautions** and be in compliance with Occupational Safety and Health Administration (OSHA) mandates and Centers for Disease Control and Prevention (CDC) guidelines.

Universal (standard) precautions is an OSHA standard requiring dental staff to treat all patients as potentially infected with a communicable disease and to wear **personal protective equipment (PPE)** when treating patients. Minimal PPE includes gloves, a face mask, eyewear or a face shield, and protective outer garments, such as scrubs or a labcoat (Figure 1-5).

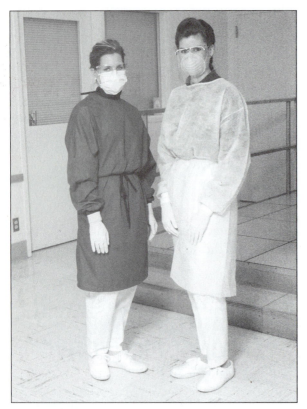

Figure 1-5 Universal (standard) precautions include the wearing of PPE: gloves, masks, eyewear, and outer clinical attire.

■ TYPES OF GLOVES USED IN DENTISTRY

Gloves are the single most important PPE component in controlling the spread of infectious disease between the dental health care worker and the patient. The dental assistant is required to wear gloves during all dental patient care procedures involving direct hand contact with saliva, blood, or other body fluids; gloving is also required when handling items contaminated with body fluids or other potentially infectious materials (OPIMs).

The dental assistant must complete proper handwashing technique before donning (putting on) and doffing (removing) gloves. For detailed information and instructions about proper handwashing technique, refer to Chapter 2: Disease Prevention in the Dental Office in *Safety Standards and Infection Control for Dental Assistants* (by E. Dietz-Bourguignon, 2002, Clifton Park, NY: Thomson Delmar Learning).

The dental assistant should be familiar with the different types of gloves available to the dental profession, their uses, their advantages, and their disadvantages. Gloves are available in a variety of sizes, from extra small to extra large, and must be made available to employees (at the employer's expense) in sizes that reasonably fit.

Disposable (Nonsterile) Examination Gloves

Disposable examination gloves are intended for single-procedure use and should be appropriately discarded following the conclusion of each chairside procedure. This includes when working with dental materials at chairside (such as mixing cements or dental impression materials) and when performing laboratory procedures such as disinfecting impressions or dental prostheses. The most common types of disposable gloves are made of either vinyl or latex (Figure 1-6).

Examination gloves are supplied nonsterilized, and most manufacturers make them equally suited to either the right or left hand. Though latex examination gloves are the most commonly used type in dentistry, vinyl gloves have come to replace latex where hand irritations (usually called contact dermatitis) are present.

Overgloves

Overgloves, intended for one-time use, are made of inexpensive clear plastic and are often referred to as food-handler's gloves. The

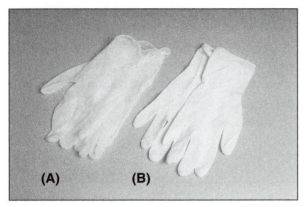

Figure 1-6 Examination gloves made of (A) vinyl and (B) latex.

overglove (Figure 1-7) is so named because it is placed over the treatment glove for temporary use, then removed when chairside duties are resumed on the same patient. Overgloves are not a suitable replacement for latex or vinyl examination gloves.

Common instances when an overglove might be worn by the dental assistant are when making chart notations, when making a denture or orthodontic appliance adjustment in the laboratory, or when taking a telephone call.

Sterile Gloves

Sterile gloves are intended for single use during oral surgery and extensive periodontal surgical procedures. They are packaged presterilized and labeled for left and right hands.

Nitrile Utility Gloves

Nitrile utility gloves are intended for multiple use and are to be worn during treatment room disinfection, instrument scrubbing and preparation, and other nontreatment procedures. Protective, heavy nitrile gloves (Figure 1-8) are puncture resistant, autoclavable, and reusable. Each staff member should have a pair of utility gloves designated with his or her name.

Nitrile gloves are not to be confused with or substituted for the less expensive household cleaning gloves sold in grocery or hardware stores.

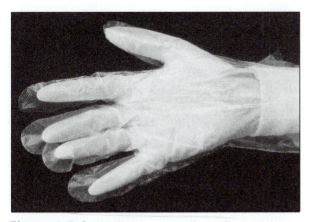

Figure 1-7 Overgloves are slipped on over examination gloves for brief activities, such as opening drawers or making chart notes. The overgloves are then removed when the original duty or procedure is resumed.

(Courtesy of Biotrol, Louisville, KY.)

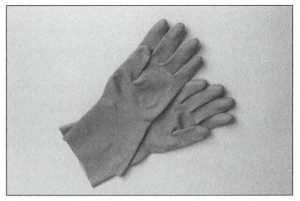

Figure 1-8 Utility gloves are worn by the dental assistant during infection control and instrument-processing procedures.

■ MASKS

Surgical face masks (Figure 1-9) must be worn when splashing or spattering of blood, saliva, or other body fluids is likely. The CDC guidelines recommend that surgical disposable masks be replaced between patients or during extended procedures when the mask becomes visibly wet or soiled with bioburden (saliva, blood, or related body fluids).

Most masks are formfitting over the bridge of the nose to minimize fogging and to fit under prescription eyewear or goggles. Commercially available styles of face masks include preformed dome-shaped masks, pliable pleated masks, and mask-eyewear combinations with elastic strap and tieback options. Masks made of glass fiber mat and synthetic fiber mat provide the highest filtration rate. The FDA recommends that surgical masks have a 95 percent or greater bacterial filtration efficiency.

The dental assistant should avoid handling the body of the mask, instead handling the mask at the periphery (edge). The assistant should also refrain from pulling the mask down to rest against his or her neck because the patient's bioburden on the outside of the mask could inadvertently contact the dental assistant's skin.

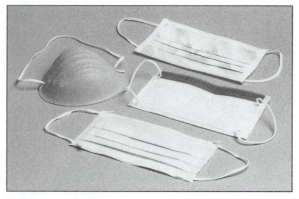

Figure 1-9 Masks are available in a variety of styles, including dome and pleated.

■ EYEWEAR

Protective eyewear is also OSHA mandated as part of PPE. Protective eyewear is designed to safeguard the eyes from diseases such as herpes simplex viruses and *Staphylococcus aureus*; eyewear also protects against contact with caustic chemicals, radiographic solutions, dental laboratory materials, and flying particulates, including pieces of scrap amalgam and tooth fragments.

The dental assistant may wear goggles (Figure 1-10A), eyeglasses with side shields (Figure 1-10B), or a plastic face shield for eye protection (Figure 1-10C). Goggles must have both front and side shields for use during exposure-prone procedures. Goggles, available with or without prescription lenses, provide the highest level of protection against front and side splashes and impacts.

Nonprescription over-the-counter glasses or prescription glasses with side shields also offer some degree of protection and often have desirable features such as replaceable lenses (in case of scratching), antifogging properties, and heat tolerance to allow autoclaving.

Chin-length face shields, which should be worn in combination with a face mask to reduce exposure to blood, saliva, or other body fluids, may be worn instead of goggles or glasses. If a face shield is used to protect against damage from solid projectiles, the protective eyewear should meet the American National Standards Institute (ANSI) Occupational and Educational Eye and Face Protection Standard and must be clearly marked as such.

Eyewear must be thoroughly washed with soap and hot water and rinsed well after each patient. Eyewear may be decontaminated and disinfected using a spray-wipe-spray method before reuse. The dental assistant should exercise

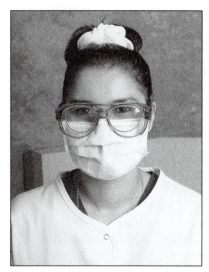

Figure 1-10A The dental assistant wears goggles and a pleated face mask.

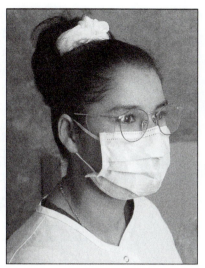

Figure 1-10B The dental assistant wears prescription eyeglasses with clear plastic side shields and a pleated mask.

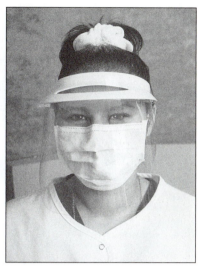

Figure 1-10C The dental assistant wears a chin-length face shield and a pleated mask.

extreme care to ensure that residual disinfectant is thoroughly removed before placing the glasses, goggles, or face shield near his or her eyes.

■ SCRUBS OR DISPOSABLE PROTECTIVE OUTER GARMENTS

Scrubs or protective outer garments must also be worn by the dental assistant when contact with spray, splashes, or body fluids can be reasonably anticipated to contaminate the torso, forearms, or lap. Suitable protective garments (worn over street clothes, undergarments, or the clinic uniform as a protective outer layer) prevent organisms on nonclinical attire from shedding into ambient air over patients with open tissues. Protective garments should be long sleeved and high necked and be free of ornamentation such as buttons or jewelry.

For routine dental procedures, disposable dental gowns (Figure 1-11) are worn once and discarded. They must be properly discarded and replaced if they become visibly contaminated, soiled, or wet.

Reusable cotton or cotton-polyester laboratory coats, clinic jackets, aprons, scrubs, or gowns, donned at the beginning of the treatment day, are acceptable alternatives to disposable protective garments. The dental assistant may not wear these articles of clothing to and from the office, outside the office, when leaving the office for lunch, or when running errands.

Laundering of Reusable PPE

Reusable protective garments may not be laundered by employees in their home laundry with their own personal clinic attire or with other family members' clothing.

OSHA's Bloodborne Pathogens Standard clearly states that laundering of protective

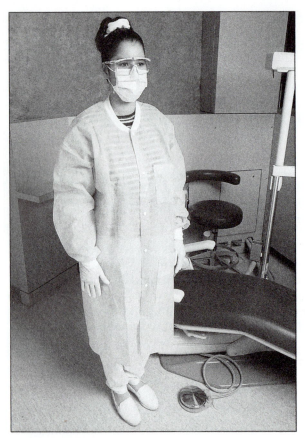

Figure 1-11 The dental assistant wears complete PPE, including disposable outer garments.

garments is the responsibility of the employer and prohibits contaminated clothing and linens from being laundered by employees in their homes. Instead, protective garment laundry must be done either on-site in the office or through a commercial laundering service or dry cleaner, provided that universal (standard) precautions are applied and PPE is in place.

The standard laundry cycle recommended by detergent and machine manufacturers is considered sufficient for decontaminating reusable clinic attire.

Unless the laundry service employees practice universal (standard) precautions in handling all laundry, contaminated laundry transported away from the practice for laundering must be packaged in leak-proof bags appropriately marked or labeled with the universal biohazard symbol.

■ IMPORTANCE OF INFECTION CONTROL AND ASEPSIS IN THE DENTAL OFFICE LABORATORY

For many years, asepsis in the dental office laboratory was often overlooked. More recently, controlling cross–contamination in the laboratory area has become equally as important as disease containment in treatment rooms. It is most often the duty of the dental assistant to implement and follow these procedures in the dental laboratory.

The CDC guidelines specifically direct that blood and saliva should be thoroughly and carefully cleaned from laboratory supplies and materials that have been used in the mouth (e.g., impression materials, bite registration), especially before polishing and grinding intraoral devices. Materials, impressions, and intraoral appliances should be cleaned and disinfected before being handled, adjusted, or sent to a commercial dental laboratory. These items should also be cleaned and disinfected when returned from the outside laboratory.

A chemical germicide that is registered with the U.S. Environmental Protection Agency (EPA) as a hospital disinfectant and that has a label claim for mycobactericidal (e.g., tuberculocidal) activity is preferred because mycobacteria represent one of the most resistant groups of microorganisms; therefore, germicides that are effective against mycobacteria are also effective against other bacterial and viral pathogens.

■ APPROPRIATE PPE IN THE LABORATORY

As when working at chairside with dental materials, when working in the dental laboratory, on dental impressions, or on prosthetic or orthodontic cases, the dental assistant must employ universal (standard) precautions. Wearing PPE not only aids in prevention of disease transmission, it also provides additional protection for the assistant against inhaling dangerous substances such as pumice and glutaraldehyde fumes or from sustaining accidental splatters, burns, or injuries that may result from flying objects such as tooth fragments or pieces of acrylic.

■ COMMUNICATION WITH THE COMMERCIAL DENTAL LABORATORY

Communication between a dental office and the commercial dental laboratory regarding handling and decontamination of dental impressions, appliances, and prostheses supplies is of the utmost importance. This communication most often is the responsibility of the dental assistant under the direction of the dentist.

Log and Track Laboratory Cases

In addition to maintaining asepsis of cases, the dental assistant must manage the flow of dental cases in and out of the office by maintaining a tracking system as to the type and nature of laboratory cases, the name of the patient, the date sent out, anticipated due date, and information about the status of the case.

A dental laboratory prescription, sometimes referred to as a work order, is written in duplicate: One copy goes to the laboratory with the case and the other is retained in the patient's chart. The prescription's dual parts are usually labeled "lab copy" and "office copy" or "doctor's copy."

To maintain current information on the status of all laboratory cases, it is helpful to set up a dental laboratory tracking system to enable the dentist and chairside assistant to know at any given time the location and status of every laboratory case sent out of the office.

This tracking system may be a notebook, a dry-wipe board in the office laboratory, or a program logged into the practice's computer database (Table 1-2).

It is also essential that the dental assistant keep a schedule of the required number of turnaround working days required by each respective laboratory to complete the procedure requested and to entrust the office manager to schedule the patient accordingly for subsequent, sequential appointments, if necessary.

It is beneficial to the practice that one dental assistant be charged with the responsibility of tracking and maintaining the status on laboratory cases; a backup staff member should have training as well.

DID YOU KNOW?

The clinician must allow sufficient time when setting up appointments for the laboratory to complete the work and return it to the office prior to the patient's next scheduled appointment.

Patient's Name	Date Sent Out	Laboratory	Work Ordered	Date Needed	Date Returned	Patient's Appointment Date
Mary Smith	10/3	Smile Dental	PFG four-unit bridge	10/17	10/15	10/24
Harold Roberts	10/5	Dental Works	FU/FL denture	10/12	10/10	11/3
Ralph Garcia	10/7	Dental Works	PU metal framework	10/18	10/17	10/20

PFG = porcelain fused to gold; FU/FL = full upper/full lower; PU = partial denture.

Table 1-2 Sample Laboratory Tracking Form

Most dental laboratories provide their own printed prescription pads for convenience. The information in Box 1-1 should appear on the outgoing laboratory prescription.

Management of Outgoing Laboratory Cases

Prior to sending out a case, the dental assistant must carefully disinfect, dry, wrap, and mark the impression, prosthesis, or appliance for shipment or pick-up. The laboratory prescription is completed with instructions for the laboratory technician.

- Patient's name (or sometimes a patient's case number or Social Security number)
- Type of service, prosthesis, or appliance required
- Type of material required, such as porcelain or metal
- Shade (tooth color) required by the dentist to match the patient's original or existing dentition and a mold number for denture teeth
- Date required for the case to be returned to the office (usually one to two days prior to the patient's reappointment time)
- Dentist's name, address, telephone number, license number, and signature or initials

Often, a member of the dental staff may write dental laboratory work orders and sign the dentist's name or initials, as directed by the dentist.

Box 1-1 Outgoing Laboratory Prescription Information

It is also helpful when communicating with commercial dental laboratories to include a laboratory asepsis form (Box 1-2), which ensures accountability in infection control practices and procedures for both the dental office and the laboratory. The dental assistant or office manager should store a copy in the practice's office manual or hazard communication manual.

This form will help the dental assistant keep track of incoming and outgoing laboratory cases. These completed records should be kept on file as a permanent part of the practice's infection control program.

■ IMPRESSIONS AND OUTGOING CASES

In accordance with CDC and OSHA guidelines, our office uses _____ for _____ minutes prior to handling or pouring models and impressions. We do this to prevent cross-contamination to laboratory personnel, to our patients, or to ourselves.

■ INCOMING CASES

We use _____ to disinfect/sterilize cases returning from the dental laboratory for _____ minutes prior to placing prostheses in the mouth. We do this to prevent cross-contamination from laboratory personnel, patients, and ourselves.

_____   _____
Doctor's Signature   Date

Box 1-2 Laboratory Asepsis Form

Management of Incoming Laboratory Cases

When a case comes in from the commercial laboratory, the dental assistant opens the box, noting the condition of the contents, the patient's name, and the type of laboratory work completed.

Incoming commercial laboratory materials, impressions, and intraoral appliances should be cleaned and disinfected before being handled, adjusted, or inserted into a patient's mouth. These items should also be cleaned and disinfected when returned from the dental laboratory and before placement in the patient's mouth.

The CDC requires that a chemical germicide be used that is EPA approved as a hospital disinfectant and that has a label claim for mycobactericidal activity.

The dental assistant should discard packaging materials immediately upon opening. To reduce the likelihood of cross-contamination, laboratory packing materials should not be saved and reused.

When the laboratory case is returned, it should be compared to the original work order or prescription for accuracy and quality. The returned case will include a copy of the prescription, which the office manager files to later compare to the monthly statements sent by the various laboratories with which the doctor works.

■ DISINFECTION OF DENTAL LABORATORY AREAS, WORK SURFACES, AND PRODUCTION AREAS

When working in the dental laboratory area, all counters and work surfaces must be kept clean and free of debris daily. The dental assistant should use the same environmental disinfection techniques as in the dental treatment rooms. The technique called spray-wipe-spray is detailed in Chapter 9: Environmental Surface and Equipment Asepsis in *Safety Standards and Infection Control for Dental Assistants* (by E. Dietz-Bourguignon, 2002, Clifton Park, NY: Thomson Delmar Learning). If unfamiliar with this technique, the dental assistant is advised to review this chapter.

Large sheets of paper work well as a surface barrier. These must be disposed of immediately after use. Any instruments, attachments, items, or materials used with new prostheses or appliances should be maintained separately from those to be used with prostheses or appliances that have already been inserted into the mouth and are thus contaminated. This separation procedure includes separate pumice pans for new and existing prostheses as well as separate polishing burrs.

Disinfection of Laboratory Pumice

If contaminated pumice is used to polish an immediate denture, the possibility exists for a potential infectious fungal, bacterial, or viral infection to be transmitted into open wounds (sockets), cross-contaminating patients.

When adjusting any removable appliance or prosthesis, the operator should wear protective gloves, mask, and eyewear to avoid contacting potentially infectious splatter, which will reduce the likelihood of cross-contamination. To protect patients, the dental assistant disinfects a fresh amount of pumice to create a slurry with a 1 : 10 mixture of chlorine bleach and water or other recommended disinfectant.

Some practices find it helpful to use cost-effective, disposable fast-food containers or grocery store Styrofoam trays. The dental assistant writes the patient's name on the pan and places a brush wheel or rag wheel in each pan for one-time use with each patient's labortory case.

Disinfection of Brush Wheels and Rag Wheels

Following each use, the dental assistant washes reusable rag wheels, then places them into a canister to be sterilized by steam under pressure. The canister tops should be loose to allow a free flow of the sterilant. Rag wheels may also be washed, rinsed, bagged, and cycled through the autoclave.

Rag wheels should not be cycled through a chemical vapor sterilizer because this process may burn the cloth portion.

A fresh wheel should be used for polishing each prosthesis or appliance. Disposable buffing wheels are a suggested alternative to reusable rag wheels. Brush wheels should be disinfected at least daily.

Disinfection of Miscellaneous Chairside Laboratory Items

Miscellaneous laboratory items used at chairside that cannot withstand sterilization or that may not fit inside a sterilizer also require disinfection. Articulators, facebows, plane guides, Boley gauges, torches, and shade guides can become contaminated with saliva.

The dental assistant should scrub them with an iodine-containing disinfectant, alternately spraying the instrument with the disinfectant, maintaining wetness for at least 2 minutes. Then the assistant wipes them dry.

If iodophors are used to disinfect shade guides, the dental assistant should wipe them with water or alcohol following exposure time to remove any residual disinfectant. If glutaraldehyde or phenolics are used on any of the above items that may come into contact with mucous membranes or skin, they must be thoroughly rinsed afterward.

■ SHELF LIFE AND INVENTORY ORDER/SUPPLY

The investment in dental materials and supplies in a dental office is substantial. Thus, the dental assistant should make every effort to avoid wasting materials. The dental assistant or office manager usually assigned the task of supply inventory and reorder should be familiar with the amounts of dental materials used and order from the dental supplier accordingly.

More specifically, ordering in large quantities may keep the per-unit cost down and appear to save the practice money; however, if items are ordered in too great a quantity, the **shelf life** (the amount of time a dental material is usable, prior to the expiration date marked on the packaging or label) may expire on consumable products before they are used. Also, the office may have insufficient storage space or refrigeration space to adequately handle large items purchased in bulk. This is expensive and wasteful to the practice.

On the other hand, items consumed quickly may require too frequent ordering or may cause the practice to run out of a material when the patient is scheduled for a procedure requiring that item.

To save embarrassment to the practice, in addition to having to reschedule the patient, the wise dental assistant or office manager always checks ahead of time to ensure that a sufficient quantity of a product or material is fresh and in stock prior to confirming that patient's appointment. Thus, in some instances, the practice may take advantage of bulk ordering of high-use items or those which do not take large storage space or require refrigeration.

■ Critical Thinking Questions

1. Why is knowledge of dental properties important to the dental assistant?

2. What does the term universal (standard) precautions mean, and why is it important to all members of the clinical dental team?

3. What is the single most important component of PPE?

4. Why is it important for the dental assistant or office manager to be familiar with dental material supply ordering and inventory management?

CHAPTER 1: POSTTEST

Instructions: For each of the following select the answer that most accurately completes the question or statement.

1. Saliva plays a role in the increase of oral acidity.
   A. True
   B. False

2. _____ is any push or pull on an object; the result is resistance.
   A. Stress
   B. Strain
   C. Force
   D. Cohesion

3. The ability of a material to withstand forces of tensile stress without failing or becoming altered is called
   A. malleability
   B. tensile strength
   C. bruxism
   D. ductility

4. Dimensional change occurs in dental materials for a variety of reasons, including all of the following *except*
   A. spatulation process
   B. setting process
   C. exposure to heat or cold associated with storage prior to activation
   D. exposure to foods or drink

5. Microleakage due to recurrent decay and dental sensitivity is the primary reason dental restorations must be removed and replaced.
   A. True
   B. False

6. Mechanical retention requires a chemical reaction between the tooth surface and the dental material.
   A. True
   B. False

7. Thermal expansion occurs when the dental material is subjected to heat: The dental material shrinks, then expands when the heat source is removed.
   A. True
   B. False

8. Universal (standard) precautions are an OSHA standard requiring dental staff to treat all patients as potentially infected with a communicable disease.
   A. True
   B. False

9. Minimal PPE required when working with dental materials at chairside includes all of the following *except*
   A. gloves
   B. face masks
   C. eyewear
   D. protective outer wear such as a labcoat or scrubs
   E. respirator masks

10. _____ are the single most important PPE component in controlling the spread of infectious disease between the dental health care worker and the patient.
    A. Face shields
    B. Masks
    C. Eyewear
    D. Gloves
    E. Protective outer wear such as scrubs or a lab coat

11. All of the following statements are true of nitrile utility gloves *except*
    A. They are intended for multiple use and are to be worn during treatment room disinfection and instrument scrubbing.
    B. They are autoclavable and reusable.
    C. They are prepackaged left/right fitted and are presterilized.
    D. They should not be substituted for less expensive household cleaning gloves sold in retail stores.

12. Wearing PPE in the dental laboratory provides the dental assistant with additional protection against all of the following *except*
    A. prevention of disease transmission
    B. inhaling dangerous or toxic substances
    C. unplanned pregnancy
    D. burns
    E. injuries from flying objects

13. Laboratory supplies, materials, and appliances must be thoroughly and carefully cleaned because:
    A. The CDC guidelines require it.
    B. Blood and saliva from the mouth contain contaminants.
    C. Commercial laboratories do not generally clean or disinfect prostheses or appliances before returning them.
    D. A and B only

14. Prior to sending out a laboratory case, the dental assistant should complete all of the following steps *except*
    A. Carefully disinfect, dry, wrap, and mark the impression or prosthesis for shipment or pickup.
    B. Complete a separate laboratory bill for the patient.
    C. Check to ensure the patient's name or patient number is included wit the case.
    D. Enter all necessary information into the office's laboratory case tracking system.
    E. Check to ensure the laboratory prescription is completed with instructions for the laboratory technician.

15. To save money, the dental assistant should save, recycle, and reuse laboratory packaging materials.
    A. True
    B. False

16. Ideally, one dental assistant should be responsible for maintaining the dental laboratory case tracking system in the office.
    A. True
    B. False

17. When ordering and maintaining dental supply inventory, the dental assistant or office manager should take into account all of the following factors *except*
    A. cost
    B. storage space
    C. shelf life
    D. rate of usage
    E. rebates and premiums offered by the dental supplier

18. Miscellaneous laboratory items used at chairside that cannot withstand sterilization or that may not fit inside a sterilizer require disinfection.
    A. True
    B. False

19. Articulators, facebows, plane guides, Boley gauges, torches, and shade guides that become contaminated with saliva can be disinfected using
    A. Lysol
    B. rubbing alcohol
    C. an iodine-containing disinfectant and then wiping dry
    D. household bleach

20. The CDC requires that a chemical germicide be used that is EPA approved as a hospital disinfectant and that has a label claim for mycobactericidal activity.
    A. True
    B. False

Cements
and Liners

To be loyal to my employer, my calling, and myself.

To develop initiative—having the courage to assume responsibility and the imagination to create ideas and develop them.

To be prepared to visualize, take advantage of, and fulfill the opportunities of my calling.

LEARNING OBJECTIVES

Upon completion of this chapter the student should be able to:

1. Describe the role and duties of the dental assistant in the use, instrumentation, manipulation, application, and clean-up procedures required when using a calcium hydroxide liner.

2. Describe the role and duties of the dental assistant in the use, instrumentation, manipulation, application, and clean-up procedures required when using a cavity varnish.

3. Describe the role and duties of the dental assistant in the use, instrumentation, manipulation, application, and clean-up procedures required when using resin cement.

4. Describe the role and duties of the dental assistant in the use, instrumentation, manipulation, and application of acid etch and bonding agents.

KEY TERMS

acid etch technique
activator
basic set-up
bonding agent
calcium hydroxide

cavity varnish
direct pulp cap
indirect pulp cap
initiator
resin cement

■ Introduction

Calcium hydroxide cavity liner, cavity varnish, resin cement, and acid etch with bonding agents are preliminary restorative materials used at chairside prior to placing a permanent restoration. The chairside dental assistant works with the dentist in the preparation, manipulation, mixing, placement, and clean-up of these materials. All preliminary restorative dental materials have specific uses, advantages, and disadvantages, (see Table 2-1).

Material	Use	Advantages	Disadvantages
Calcium hydroxide	Low-strength liner used for direct and indirect pulp capping	Ease of manipulation Little or no odor Protects pulp from bacteria and irritants Soothing effect on pulp Aids in formation of secondary dentin	None
Cavity varnish	Cavity liner, dentinal tubule sealer	Fast-drying Requires no mixing prior to placement Prevents acids in dental cements from entering dentinal tubules Prevents tooth discoloration Nonirritating to pulp, nonacidic	Requires two applications Evaporates very quickly Unpleasant taste/odor
Resin cement	Permanent cementation of cast crowns, bridges, inlays, onlays, endodontic posts, orthodontic bands, and composite and resin-bonded bridges	Radiopaque Provides sufficient strength and wear resistance required for cementation Insoluble in saliva Some contain fluoride Does not adhere to ceramic or metal	Causes irritation to the pulp Bonding required (extra chairside time)
Acid etch	Increases/enhances bonding strength between tooth surface and restorations of sealants, veneers, amalgam restorations, and composite resins	Increases retention Reduces marginal leakage	Requires extra chairside steps (bonding)

Table 2-1 Preliminary Dental Restorative Materials

These materials are mixed upon the direction and preference of the dentist. The dental assistant must follow the manufacturer's instructions when working with all materials. As when working with any material used during an invasive dental procedure, chairside personnel must wear the necessary PPE.

■ Calcium Hydroxide

Calcium hydroxide is applied by the dentist in thin "smear" layers to the walls and floor of the deepest portion of the cavity preparation to protect the pulp from bacteria and irritants. It is not applied beyond the dentinoenamel junction of the preparation because it would eventually dissolve, leading to marginal leakage (Figure 2-1).

Use

Calcium hydroxide is used as a low-strength cavity liner placed under permanent dental restorations, such as composites and amalgam.

Calcium hydroxide is used for **indirect** or **direct pulp capping** because it has a therapeutic or soothing effect on the dental pulp. Calcium hydroxide also aids in the formation of secondary dentin, also known as reparative dentin.

Composition

Calcium hydroxide is supplied in a variety of forms: powder/liquid (aqueous: containing water, formed by mixing distilled water with calcium hydroxide powder), a two-paste system (nonaqueous: containing calcium hydroxide and zinc oxide powder suspended in a chloroform solution of natural or synthetic resin), or a single-paste system (urethane dimethacrylate). The form most often used in general practice is the two-paste system, supplied in tubes: One is the catalyst and the other is the base (Figure 2-2).

Light-cured calcium hydroxide, composed of urethane dimethacrylate (similar to a composite), is also supplied in a single paste; it requires a blue cure light for a quick-setting reaction. This form of calcium hydroxide is considered more stable than the two-paste system and does not harm the dental pulp.

Properties

Calcium hydroxide provides low thermal conductivity but is not usually used to provide thermal protection to the pulp.

Some types of calcium hydroxide do not provide sufficient hardness or strength to

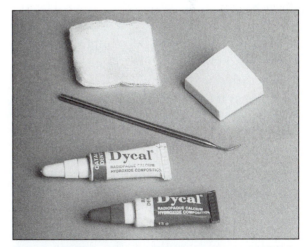

Figure 2-2 Calcium hydroxide liner supplied in a two-paste system with applicator, mixing pad, and 2 × 2 gauze.

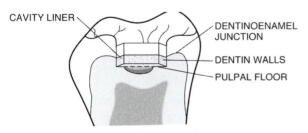

CAVITY LINER
DENTINOENAMEL JUNCTION
DENTIN WALLS
PULPAL FLOOR

Figure 2-1 Application of a cavity liner.

warrant their use alone as a base in a deep cavity. If the dentist determines that an insulating medium is required, such as in an especially deep restoration, a cement base will also be indicated (see Chapter 3). Thus, calcium hydroxide liner is usually overlaid with a stronger cement to provide protection against condensation and mastication forces.

Calcium hydroxide liner also has bacteriostatic properties; that is, it keeps bacteria from actively spreading.

Mixing/Manipulation

The dental assistant mixes the two-paste system on a small paper mixing pad provided by the manufacturer. One drop is dispensed equally from each tube onto the paper mixing pad in close proximity to but not touching the other.

The dentist indicates to the dental assistant when the calcium hydroxide mix should begin. Mixing can be done with either a small metal cement spatula or the ball applicator instrument provided by the manufacturer.

Mixing takes place when the dental assistant incorporates the two drops together. The result is a consistent-colored fluid mix with no streaks; mixing should be completed within 10–15 seconds.

When the mix is complete, the dental assistant masses it together in the center of the pad and brings the pad close to the patient's chin, out of his or her line of vision, and passes the ball applicator to the dentist. The dentist then "drags" the applicator through the mix and places the calcium hydroxide liner to form a smear layer in the cavity preparation.

When the calcium hydroxide liner application has been completed, the dentist hands the applicator instrument back to the assistant, who then wipes the applicator and mixing spatula (if used) dry with a 2 × 2 gauze sponge. This prevents the liner material from drying or caking on the metal instrument(s) and makes clean-up easier at the conclusion of the procedure.

■ Cavity Varnish

Cavity varnish is an amber-colored liquid resin applied by the dentist to the prepared dentin; the manufacturer also supplies a liquid solvent, of which the dental assistant occasionally adds small amounts to the varnish as it thickens over time or in cleaning instruments that may have become sticky from contacting the varnish directly.

Use

Cavity varnish is applied, often in several layers (place, air-dry, place again, being careful not to cross-contaminate), to the enamel and dentin walls up to the cavosurface margin of the tooth preparation (Figure 2-3) to seal the dentinal tubules exposed during an amalgam cavity preparation (Figure 2-4).

Cavity varnish evaporates quickly, leaves a thin film, and acts as a semipermeable membrane to prevent the passage of acids from cement along the dentinal tubules to the pulp. Cavity varnish also reduces the number of metallic ions penetrating the tissues of the dentin and enamel, thus minimizing the discoloration of the tooth structure next to the restoration.

DID YOU KNOW?

Calcium hydroxide is very moisture-sensitive. Humidity from the air or exposure to water will accelerate the hardening of the mix.

Calcium Hydroxide Two-Paste System

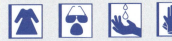

ARMAMENTARIUM

- **Basic set-up** (mouth mirror, explorer, cotton pliers, and sometimes a periodontal probe)
- Calcium hydroxide tubes: one catalyst, one base
- Paper mixing pad
- Small (metal) cement mixing spatula (optional)
- Small ball applicator instrument (miniature ball burnisher)
- 2 × 2 gauze sponges

PROCEDURE

1. Dispense (gently squeeze) one small drop each of the catalyst and base next to each other, but not touching, onto the paper mixing pad.
2. Use a 2 × 2 gauze sponge to wipe off excess liner material from each of the tubes before replacing the corresponding caps. (Note that each cap is color coded to its corresponding tube.) Replace caps.
3. Using a circular motion, incorporate the two liquids thoroughly until a uniform consistency and color are reached (10–15 seconds).
4. Use a clean 2 × 2 gauze sponge to wipe excess material from the spatula or small ball applicator instrument.
5. Pass the small ball applicator instrument to the dentist and hold the paper mixing pad close to the patient's chin, out of his or her line of vision.
6. Use a fresh 2 × 2 gauze sponge to remove excess liner material from the applicator, as directed by the dentist, between applications.
7. At completion of the application, receive the small ball applicator from the dentist, wipe any excess liner from the applicator, and return the materials to the instrument tray or work surface.
8. Tear off and fold closed the top layer of the contaminated mixing pad and dispose of it. (Folding the paper helps prevent further contamination of the worksite and keeps the material from inadvertently sticking to other items on the instrument tray.)

Special Considerations

- Do not allow contents of the tubes to touch prior to mixing. (This is to prevent contamination.)
- Always wipe mixed material from instruments immediately after application to prevent caking.
- Always wear PPE when working at chairside.
- Maintain and work in a clean, dry, aseptic field.
- Clean and disinfect the work area at the conclusion of the procedure, after dismissing the patient.
- Always follow OSHA regulations and CDC recommendations to help prevent the spread of bloodborne diseases and to protect dental personnel.

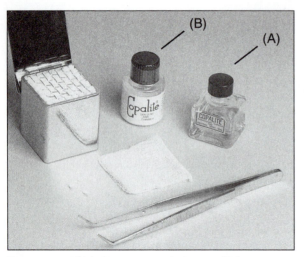

Figure 2-3 (A) Cavity varnish and (B) solvent are used to seal dentin tubules. The cotton pellet is dipped into the varnish with cotton pliers, then dabbed on the inside of the bottle prior to removing it to prevent oversaturation of the pellet, which may cause dripping.

To summarize, cavity varnish is used to:
- Prevent tooth sensitivity by sealing dentinal tubules exposed during cavity preparation.
- Prevent acids in dental cements from entering the dentinal tubules.
- Prevent tooth discoloration by impeding metallic ions from penetrating dentinal tubules.

The indications for application of cavity varnish depend upon the type of restoration indicated and whether a cement base is to be

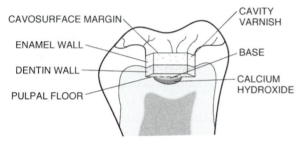

Figure 2-4 Cavity varnish applied after calcium hydroxide liner and cement base.

applied. In general, cavity varnish is applied prior to the placement of zinc phosphate cement, amalgam, or gold foil restorations. Cavity varnish is applied after calcium hydroxide liner.

Composition

Varnish is a natural gum or a (copal) solution. Copal varnish contains organic solvents such as ether, acetone, or chloroform. It is used for crown preparations or under amalgam restorations because some forms of varnish interfere with polymerization of acrylic and resin restorative materials. If left uncovered, it will rapidly evaporate.

Universal varnishes, also called synthetic varnishes, do not have organic solvents and may be used under all restorations, including composite restorations.

The solvent is a volatile organic liquid such as acetone, chloroform, or ether and is subject to evaporation if left uncovered.

Properties

Cavity varnish does not provide strength or thermal insulation to the dental pulp. Varnish is insoluble in the oral cavity; its primary function is to reduce leakage around the margins of dental restorations, preventing a phenomenon called microleakage.

The solvent within the varnish acts as a vehicle to carry the resin or polymer to the tooth preparation and then evaporates, leaving behind a resin or polymer film. Because the film is porous, the varnish is usually applied twice (within 20–30 seconds) to ensure a more uniform coating.

Varnish adheres physically, not chemically, to the tooth surface.

Another function of cavity varnish is to prevent acids released by some dental cements from penetrating into the dentin. Cavity varnish is both nonirritating (to the pulp) and nonacidic.

Mixing/Manipulation

Because varnish is made from materials that evaporate easily, care must be taken to immediately replace the bottle cap once the amount required for the procedure has been removed from the bottle.

Often, cavity varnish is applied in two coats to provide greater protection and coverage of the dentin to prevent voids.

Cavity varnish is one of the few dental materials that does not require mixing. It is placed directly onto the exposed dentin by the dentist using a cotton pellet, applicator brush, or wire applicator loop dipped directly into the cavity varnish bottle. A second coat is usually required.

■ Resin Cement

Resin cements have a wide variety of applications in dentistry (Figure 2-5). They are supplied in a two-paste system, in a powder and liquid set, or in a premixed syringe. Sometimes resin cements are supplied with an accompanying acid etch gel or liquid; some are shaded to match the translucency of the porcelain crown, inlay, or veneer.

PRACTICE MAKES PERFECT PROCEDURE ■ 2-2

Cavity Varnish

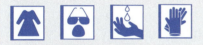

ARMAMENTARIUM
- Basic set-up (including locking cotton pliers)
- Cavity varnish and solvent (optional)
- Cotton pellets, cotton pellet dispenser/application brush or wire applicator loop
- Air-water syringe

PROCEDURE
1. Using the air-water syringe, thoroughly wash and dry the prepared tooth.
2. Grasp the locking cotton pliers, open the bottle of cavity varnish, and gently dip one cotton pellet until it is saturated with the solution. Lock the cotton pliers.
3. Dab the saturated cotton pellet on the inside of the bottle, ensuring that the excess varnish remains in the bottle and does not drip.
4. Remove the cotton pellet from the cavity varnish bottle.
5. Quickly replace the cavity varnish bottle cap (to prevent evaporation) and pass the cotton pellet secured in the locked cotton pliers to the dentist, handle first.
6. For the second application of cavity varnish, the dental assistant receives the used cotton pellet still locked in the cotton pliers, removes and discards the used pellet, selects a fresh cotton pellet, and repeats steps 4 and 5.
7. After completing the cavity varnish application, the dental assistant receives the (still) locked cotton pliers from the dentist and releases the used pellet from the pliers and discards it into a proper chairside waste receptacle; this is to prevent them from sticking to other instruments or cotton products used in the working field.
8. At clean-up, the dental assistant may use a small amount of solvent to remove excess cavity varnish from the cotton pliers.

Three types of resin cement are available: self-curing (chemical), light cured (photo), and dual cured. Dual-cured resin cements contain chemicals that self-cure (called autopolymerization) or are light cured (called photopolymerization).

Use

Resin cements can be bonded to enamel or dentin. They may be used for permanent cementation of cast metal restorations and porcelain-fused-to-resin restorations as well as for veneers, orthodontic brackets, and endodontic posts.

Self-curing resin cements are indicated for use with metal or metal combination restorations and endodontic posts; light-cured resin cements are indicated for porcelain/resin restorations, for veneers, and to cement orthodontic brackets.

Dual-cured resin cements are commonly used to lute (cement) composite or porcelain inlays, onlays, crowns, or veneers because these restorations partially transmit light (this is sometimes referred to as opaque). Cement does not illuminate through metal castings or bridges.

Composition

Resin cements are fluid composites. Resin matrices are BIS-GMA (bisphenol A-glycidyl methacrylate) or dimethacrylate resin diluted with low-viscosity monomers. Resin cements are more fluid than direct-filling composites because the number of filler particles is reduced to create low viscosity to aid cementation.

The fillers contained in resin cements are usually barium glasses, although some resin cements are filled with microscopic silica particles. Fillers make up 30–60 percent by weight of resin cement.

Properties

Many resin cements are radiopaque and provide sufficient strength and wear resistance required for cementation. Resin cements are

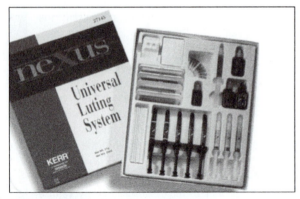

Figure 2-5 Resin cement system.

(Courtesy of Kerr Corporation.)

insoluble in saliva but are known to cause pulpal irritation; thus a protective cement is required. Additionally, some resin cements contain fluoride, which is released slowly into the oral cavity and helps prevent secondary (recurrent) caries.

Resin cements do not adhere to ceramic materials or to metal casting; thus, they must be roughened with acid etchant to produce a mechanical bonding or the tissue surfaces of ceramics must be treated with a silane coupling agent that produces a chemical bond with the resin cement. In some instances, a wire mesh or undercuts may be added to the tissue side of the prosthesis to ensure permanent retention.

Mixing/Manipulation

Self-curing resin cements are supplied with an **initiator** (a substance that contains molecules that cause or initiate a polymerization reaction) and an **activator** (a chemical, usually an amine compound, that causes initiator molecules to become active and to begin a polymerization reaction). The dental assistant mixes these two materials on a paper pad for 20–30 seconds, taking care to remove excess cement before the material is completely set; this is to prevent marginal leakage.

Light-cured resin cements are supplied in syringes and must be cured for a minimum of 40 seconds.

Dual-cured resin cements are supplied in two component systems that are mixed together for 20–30 seconds.

Once mixed, resin cement sets slowly, allowing working time to place the resin cement in the areas of the prosthesis desired and for the prosthesis to be seated properly in the oral cavity. Once the dentist is satisfied that the prosthesis is properly fitted, polished,

equilibrated, and positioned, the visible-light unit is activated to polymerize the resin cement.

■ ACID ETCH AND BONDING AGENTS

Bonding agents are also called adhesives or bonding resins. Adhesion (sticking or adhering) of dental restorative materials or restorations is achieved using an **acid etch technique** in which the tooth structure is treated with phosphoric acid. This solution roughens or etches the tooth surface and creates microscopic undercuts that enhance retention of the resin or porcelain restoration (Figure 2-6). These microscopic undercuts are referred to as chemical bond, defined earlier in this chapter.

Because marginal leakage around restorations, especially resin restorations, has been a significant concern to dentistry, the introduction of bonding agents has proven an effective way to seal resin restorations using an acid etch technique prior to placing a restoration.

Use

Bonding agents are used to increase or enhance retention between the tooth structure (enamel or dentin) and restorations such as

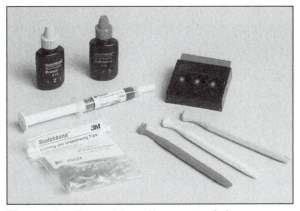

Figure 2-6 Dental bonding materials.

Resin Cement: Dual-Curing System

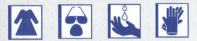

ARMAMENTARIUM

- Basic set-up
- Cotton rolls
- Air-water syringe
- Dual-system resin cement, including etchant and adhesive
- Paper mixing pad
- Stainless steel spatula
- Plastic placement instrument
- Curing light and protective shield or glasses
- 2 × 2 gauze sponges

PROCEDURE

1. Clean and dry the tooth or teeth and isolate the area with cotton rolls.
2. Pass the etchant gel or solution to the dentist.
3. Wait until the etchant has taken effect; using the air-water syringe, rinse and dry the tooth/teeth thoroughly.
4. Apply the adhesive.
5. Dispense and mix equal parts of the activator and initiator until a homogenous, creamy mixture results (30 seconds working time).
6. Transfer and hold the paper mixing pad close to the patient's chin and pass the plastic placement instrument to the dentist to place the material onto the tooth/teeth and into the restoration.
7. Provide a 2 × 2 gauze sponge for the dentist to remove any excess resin cement material.
8. Receive the plastic instrument and ready the curing light.
9. Hold the curing light and place the protective shield over the oral cavity when the light is activated (this is to prevent permanent damage to the eyes).
10. When the procedure has been completed, dismiss the patient and clean the operating area immediately. Discard disposable items appropriately.

Special Considerations

- Always wear PPE when working at chairside.
- Maintain and work in a clean, dry, aseptic field.
- Clean and disinfect the work area at the conclusion of the procedure, after dismissing the patient.
- Always follow OSHA regulations and CDC recommendations to help prevent the spread of bloodborne diseases and to protect dental personnel.

porcelain, resins, precious and nonprecious metals, composites, and amalgam. Bonding to enamel is required prior to placement of composite restoration, pit and fissure sealants, veneers, resin-cemented crowns and bridges, and orthodontic brackets.

Composition

The acid–etching process requires the use of a 30 percent to 50 percent phosphoric acid solution; the most common concentration is 37 percent. The etching liquid or gel is supplied by the manufacturer in bottles or

Application of Acid Etchant

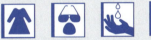

ARMAMENTARIUM

- Basic set-up
- Acid etch gel or liquid
- Isolation materials (complete dental dam set-up or cotton rolls)
- Acid etch applicator (syringe or cotton pellets)
- Dappen dish
- Air-water syringe
- Timer

PROCEDURE

1. Isolate the tooth or teeth to be acid etched.
2. Thoroughly rinse and dry the teeth to be acid etched.
3. Prepare the acid etchant material by either placing a few drops of the solution into the dappen dish and dipping a small cotton pellet into the solution or by clearing the acid etchant syringe and expressing a small amount for ready use for the dentist.
4. Pass the acid etch set-up to the dentist to apply to the teeth for 15–30 seconds (according to the manufacturer's instructions).
5. After the dentist is satisfied that the enamel or dentin is properly etched, rinse the teeth with the air-water syringe and then thoroughly dry the area for 15–30 seconds. The teeth will have a frosted appearance. The surface(s) must be kept completely dry until cementation of the prosthesis or application of the restoration or bracket is completed. Otherwise, moisture will contaminate the procedure, which must then be repeated.

Special Considerations

- Make sure the tooth is sufficiently etched for satisfactory bonding to be achieved.
- Always wear PPE when working at chairside.
- Maintain and work in a clean, dry, aseptic field.
- Clean and disinfect the work area at the conclusion of the procedure, after dismissing the patient.
- Always follow OSHA regulations and CDC recommendations to help prevent the spread of bloodborne diseases and to protect dental personnel.

syringes. Gel is the preferred form of acid etch because dentists find it easier to confine to the desired area of the tooth or teeth being treated.

Bonding agents are low-viscosity (viscous means "sticky") resins, some of which contain fillers; others contain additives with adhesive enhancers; still others contain fluoride. Bonding agents contain a dentin surface cleaner, a weak acidic solution of nitric, maleic, or EDTA (ethylenediaminetetraacetic acid). The solution may be a cleaner, a conditioner, or an etchant. Some universal bonding agent systems use etchants applicable for both enamel and dentin. These solutions remove the smear layer and produce a subtle opening of the dentinal tubules and provide etching of the surface and the dentinal tubules.

Next, a primer is applied to wet the surface of the tooth or teeth and may also potentially chemically bond to the dentin. These molecules vary by product, but include NPE, HEMA for bonding to the dentin and glutaraldehyde, and 4-META, which reacts with collagen.

Next, the bonding resin is applied to the primed tooth surface. The bonding resin consists of a low-viscosity polymerizable monomer that contains adhesive molecules.

PRACTICE MAKES PERFECT PROCEDURE ▪ 2-5

Application of Bonding Agent

ARMAMENTARIUM

- Basic set-up
- Bonding system with acid etchant, primer or tooth conditioner, adhesive
- Bonding agent applicators (disposable tips or brushes supplied by the manufacturer)
- Dappen dish
- Isolation materials (complete dental dam set-up or cotton rolls)
- Air-water syringe
- Curing light and shield
- Timer

PROCEDURE

1. If the tooth preparation is near the pulp, the dentist may request a calcium hydroxide liner or glass ionomer cement to protect and insulate the tooth.
2. The etchant is applied and rinsed, following the instructions from Practice Makes Perfect Procedure 2-4.
3. The dentist applies a primer or conditioner using a brush or an applicator when both the enamel and dentin are involved. (The purpose is to wet the dentin and penetrate the dentinal tubules.)
4. The bonding resin is applied and the curing light (with protective shield) is used to polymerize the bonding resin.
5. At the completion of the procedure, after dismissing the patient, the dental assistant disposes of the applicator tips or brushes.

Special Considerations
- Always wear PPE when working at chairside.
- Maintain and work in a clean, dry, aseptic field.
- Clean and disinfect the work area at the conclusion of procedure, after dismissing the patient.
- Always follow OSHA regulations and CDC recommendations to help prevent the spread of bloodborne diseases and to protect dental personnel.

This bonding resin wets and flows into the irregularities in the primed dentin surface to provide a mechanical bond to the tooth surface.

Properties

Low-viscosity, unfilled resin bonding agents penetrate into the microscopic tooth structure undercuts and mechanically lock into them. The restoration or restorative materials then bond to this layer. Bonding agents are either light cured or dual cured.

Mixing/Manipulation

The etchant is placed with small cotton pellets, sponges, brushes, or disposable applicators onto the tooth structure.

Bonding to dentin is more challenging because dentin has a higher moisture content and higher organic content than enamel, which can inhibit the bonding process. Because dentin is closer to the dental pulp, the dentist must take great care not to damage the pulp.

■ CRITICAL THINKING QUESTIONS

1. What is the primary use of calcium hydroxide cavity liner?
2. What are the three purposes of cavity varnish?
3. Why are resin cements formulated to set slowly?
4. What is the purpose of applying acid etch prior to using a bonding agent?

PRACTICE MAKES PERFECT
STUDENT ASSESSMENT 2-1

Calcium Hydroxide Two-Paste System

Student's Name: _____

Date: _____   Instructor: _____

Note: The blank space is provided for the instructor to check off the student's progress. The student may practice the procedure as many times as necessary before being evaluated. Some portions of the exercise may be performed on a typodont or extracted tooth or simulated in a clinical operatory. The student has successfully completed the following:

_____ Worn necessary PPE

_____ Assembled necessary armamentarium

_____ Maintained a clear, dry, aseptic working field

_____ Dispensed one small drop each of the catalyst and base onto the mixing pad, next to, but not touching, each other

_____ Used a 2 × 2 gauze sponge to wipe off excess liner material from each of the tubes before replacing the corresponding caps

_____ Replaced tube caps

_____ Used a circular motion to incorporate the two liquids thoroughly, until a uniform consistency and color were achieved (within 10–15 seconds)

_____ Used a clean 2 × 2 gauze sponge to wipe excess material from the mixing spatula or small ball applicator instrument

_____ Passed the small ball applicator instrument to the dentist and held the paper mixing pad close to the patient's chin, out of his or her line of vision

_____ Used a fresh 2 × 2 gauze sponge to remove excess liner material from the applicator, as directed by the dentist, between applications

_____ At completion of the application, received the applicator from the dentist, wiped excess liner from the applicator, and returned the materials to the instrument tray or work surface

_____ Tore off and folded closed the top layer of the contaminated mixing pad and disposed of it

_____ Replaced all items to the storage area and cleaned the work area
_____ Followed required instrument washing, disinfection, and sterilization procedures
_____ Followed OSHA guidelines and CDC recommendations to help prevent the spread of bloodborne diseases and to protect dental personnel

Comments

_____

_____

_____

_____

_____

_____

_____

Cavity Varnish

Student's Name: _____

Date: _____   Instructor: _____

Note: The blank space is provided for the instructor to check off the student's progress. The student may practice the procedure as many times as necessary before being evaluated. Some portions of the exercise may be performed on a typodont or extracted tooth or simulated in a clinical operatory. The student has successfully completed the following:

_____ Worn necessary PPE

_____ Assembled necessary armamentarium

_____ Maintained a clear, dry, aseptic working field

_____ Used the three-way syringe to thoroughly wash and dry the prepared tooth

_____ Used the locking cotton pliers to gently dip one cotton pellet completely into the cavity varnish

_____ Locked the cotton pliers to secure the pellet

_____ Dabbed the saturated cotton pellet on the inside of the bottle to ensure that the excess varnish did not drip during transfer

_____ Removed the cotton pliers and the completely moistened pellet from the cavity varnish

_____ Quickly replaced the cavity varnish bottle cap (to prevent evaporation) and passed the cotton pellet on the locked cotton pliers to the dentist, handle first

_____ Following the completion of cavity varnish application, received the used cotton pellet still locked in the cotton pliers and removed the used pellet

_____ Properly discarded and disposed of the used cotton pellet

_____ Used a small amount of solvent to remove excess cavity varnish from the cotton pliers

_____ Replaced all items to the storage area and cleaned the work area

_____ Followed required instrument washing, disinfection, and sterilization procedures

_____ Followed OSHA guidelines and CDC recommendations to help prevent the spread of bloodborne diseases and to protect dental personnel

Comments

_____

_____

_____

_____

_____

Resin Cement: Dual-Curing System

Student's Name: _____

Date: _____   Instructor: _____

Note: The blank space is provided for the instructor to check off the student's progress. The student may practice the procedure as many times as necessary before being evaluated. Some portions of the exercise may be performed on a typodont or extracted tooth or simulated in a clinical operatory. The student has successfully completed the following:

_____ Worn necessary PPE

_____ Assembled necessary armamentarium

_____ Maintained a clear, dry, aseptic working field

_____ Cleaned and dried the tooth or teeth and isolated the area with cotton rolls

_____ Passed the etchant gel or solution to the dentist

_____ Waited until the etchant took effect; rinsed and dried the tooth or teeth thoroughly

_____ Applied the adhesive

_____ Dispensed and mixed equal parts of the activator and initiator until a homogenous, creamy mixture resulted within the 30 seconds working time allotted

_____ Transferred and held the paper mixing pad close to the patient's chin and passed the plastic placement instrument to the dentist to place the material onto the tooth or teeth and into the restoration

_____ Provided a 2 × 2 gauze sponge to remove excess resin cement material

_____ Received the plastic instrument and prepared the curing light

_____ Held the curing light and placed the protective shield over the oral cavity when the light was activated to prevent permanent damage to the eyes

_____ When the procedure has been completed, dismissed the patient and cleaned the operating area immediately; discarded disposable items appropriately

_____ Replaced all items to the storage area and cleaned the work area

_____ Followed required instrument washing, disinfection, and sterilization procedures

_____ Followed OSHA guidelines and CDC recommendations to help prevent the spread of bloodborne diseases and to protect dental personnel

Comments

_____

_____

_____

_____

_____

Application of Acid Etchant

Student's Name: _____

Date: _____   Instructor: _____

Note: The blank space is provided for the instructor to check off the student's progress. The student may practice the procedure as many times as necessary before being evaluated. Some portions of the exercise may be performed on a typodont or extracted tooth or simulated in a clinical operatory. The student has successfully completed the following:

_____ Worn necessary PPE

_____ Assembled necessary armamentarium

_____ Maintained a clear, dry, aseptic working field

_____ Properly isolated the tooth or teeth to be acid etched

_____ Thoroughly rinsed and dried the teeth to be acid etched

_____ Prepared the acid etchant material by either placing a few drops of the solution into the dappen dish and dipping a small cotton pellet into the solution or clearing the acid etchant syringe and expressing a small amount for ready use for the dentist

_____ Passed the acid etch set-up to the dentist for application to the teeth for 15–30 seconds (according to the manufacturer's instructions)

_____ After the dentist was satisfied that the enamel or dentin is satisfactorily etched, rinsed the teeth with the air-water syringe and then thoroughly dried the area for 15–50 seconds

_____ Cleaned and disinfected the work area at the conclusion of the procedure, after dismissing the patient

_____ Followed required instrument washing, disinfection, and sterilization procedures

_____ Followed OSHA regulations and CDC recommendations to help prevent the spread of bloodborne diseases and to protect dental personnel

Comments

_____

_____

_____

_____

_____

Application of Bonding Agent

Student's Name: _____

Date: _____ Instructor: _____

Note: The blank space is provided for the instructor to check off the student's progress. The student may practice the procedure as many times as necessary before being evaluated. Some portions of the exercise may be performed on a typodont or extracted tooth or simulated in a clinical operatory. The student has successfully completed the following:

_____ Worn necessary PPE
_____ Assembled necessary armamentarium
_____ Maintained a clear, dry, aseptic working field
_____ Thoroughly washed and dried the area, using the air-water syringe
_____ Prepared a calcium hydroxide or glass ionomer liner, if requested by the dentist
_____ Prepared and passed the acid etch material, then passed to the dentist, following the instructions from the previous Practice Makes Perfect Procedure 2-4
_____ Assisted the dentist in application of a primer or conditioner using a brush or an applicator
_____ Assisted the dentist in application of the bonding resin and held the curing light (with protective shield) to polymerize the bonding resin
_____ At the completion of the procedure, after dismissing the patient, disposed of the applicator tips or brushes
_____ Cleaned and disinfected the work area at the conclusion of the procedure, after dismissing the patient
_____ Followed required instrument washing, disinfection, and sterilization procedures
_____ Followed OSHA regulations and CDC recommendations to help prevent the spread of bloodborne diseases and to protect dental personnel

Comments

_____
_____
_____
_____
_____

CHAPTER 2: POSTTEST

Instructions: For each of the following, select the answer that most accurately completes the question or statement.

1. All of the following are preliminary restorative materials used in preparation for placement of a permanent restoration *except*
   A. calcium hydroxide
   B. amalgam
   C. cavity varnish
   D. resin cement
   E. bonding agent

2. Calcium hydroxide liner is supplied in all of the following forms *except*
   A. one-paste
   B. two-paste
   C. powder and liquid
   D. an autopolymerizing single paste

3. Calcium hydroxide liner has bacteriostatic properties, which means it may cause bacteria to multiply.
   A. True
   B. False

4. All of the following are included in a calcium hydroxide armamentarium *except*
   A. glass mixing slab
   B. basic set-up
   C. paper mixing pad
   D. one tube each, catalyst and base
   E. small ball applicator instrument

5. At the conclusion of calcium hydroxide liner application, the dental assistant tears off and folds the top sheet from the paper mixing pad to
   A. provide extra room on the mixing pad for the next mix
   B. prevent the materials from sticking to other items on the instrument tray
   C. prevent further contamination of the worksite
   D. A and B only
   E. B and C only

6. The dental assistant should regularly add large quantities of solvent to cavity varnish to keep it diluted.
   A. True
   B. False

7. Cavity varnish is used for all of the following reasons *except*
   A. prevent tooth sensitivity by sealing dentinal tubules exposed during cavity preparation
   B. prevent acids in dental cements from entering the dentinal tubules
   C. promote the growth of secondary dentin
   D. prevent tooth discoloration by impeding metallic ions from penetrating dentinal tubules

8. Cavity varnish is routinely placed under composite restorations.
   A. True
   B. False

9. Cavity varnish is _____ in the oral cavity.
   A. soluble
   B. insoluble
   C. unstable
   D. organic

10. The solvent in cavity varnish carries the resin or polymer in the varnish to the tooth preparation and then evaporates, leaving behind a resin or polymer film.
    A. True
    B. False

11. Cavity varnish is usually applied in two coats, within _____ seconds to ensure a uniform coating and sealing of the dentinal tubules.
    A. 5–10
    B. 10–15
    C. 20–30
    D. 40–60

12. Resin cements can be bonded to which of the following natural tooth structures?
    A. enamel
    B. dentin
    C. cementum
    D. pulp
    E. A and B only
    F. C and D only

13. Self-curing resin cements are indicated for use with all of the following *except*
    A. orthodontic brackets
    B. metal restorations
    C. metal combination restorations
    D. endodontic posts

14. Light-cured resin cements are indicated for all of the following *except*
    A. porcelain/resin restorations
    B. veneers
    C. endodontic posts
    D. orthodontic brackets

15. Resin cements are more fluid than direct-filling composites because:
    A. The number of filler particles is reduced to create low viscosity to aid cementation.
    B. They are more difficult to work with.
    C. They contain more water.
    D. They absorb water from organic materials inherent in dentin.

16. Resin cements
   A. soothe the pulp
   B. cause pulpal irritation
   C. replace acid etch
   D. are soluble in saliva

17. Acid etch technique is used for all of the following applications in dental practice *except* to
   A. toughen the tooth surface
   B. create microscopic undercuts
   C. replace amalgam restorations
   D. enhance retention of resin or porcelain restorations

18. Bonding agents are an effective method of sealing resin restorations.
   A. True
   B. False

19. The most commonly used phosphoric acid in acid etch technique is a _____ concentration.
   A. 5%
   B. 10%
   C. 33%
   D. 37%
   E. 60%

20. When properly etched, the natural tooth will have a/an _____ appearance.
   A. clear
   B. opaque
   C. frosted
   D. dark

LEARNING OBJECTIVES

Upon completion of this chapter the student should be able to:

1. Describe the general types of cements used in dentistry and their specific applications.

2. Describe the role and duties of the dental assistant in the use, instrumentation, manipulation, application, and clean-up procedures required when using zinc phosphate cement.

3. Describe the role and duties of the dental assistant in the use, instrumentation, manipulation, application, and clean-up procedures required when using zinc oxide eugenol cement.

4. Describe the role and duties of the dental assistant in the use, instrumentation, manipulation, application, and clean-up procedures required when using polycarboxylate cement.

5. Describe the role and duties of the dental assistant in the use, instrumentation, manipulation, application, and clean-up procedures required when using glass ionomer cement.

KEY TERMS

exothermic reaction
glass ionomer cement
lute/luting
polycarboxylate cement
(zinc polyacrylate
cement)

zinc oxide eugenol (ZOE)
cement

■ INTRODUCTION

Cements are widely used in dentistry for a variety of applications, including but not limited to chairside restorative, prosthodontic, and orthodontic procedures. In general, cements are supplied as a powder and liquid, a two-paste system, or a capsule or in a premixed dispensing syringe. The method used in a dental office is generally dictated by economic factors. Dental cements are mixed at chairside by the dental assistant and, when prepared, passed to the dentist for direct application into the patient's oral cavity.

The consistency of dental cements may range from a pliable liquid to a thick, putty-like paste. Dental cements set, or "cure," either using a self-curing (autocuring) process (a chemical reaction between two materials) or by light curing. Self-cured cements are usually hand mixed by the dental assistant. Light-cured cements are easier to work with because they afford the operator the flexibility of additional manipulation and working time in the mouth prior to initiating the final cure.

The dental assistant should be aware that some light-cured dental cements may be affected by ambient (outside) forms of light, especially by halogen or fluorescent light in the treatment room. The dental assistant should be aware of this when setting out materials ahead of time for a cementation procedure.

Dental cements are used alone or in combination with other dental materials, such as amalgam or composite restorations, veneers, single-unit or multiple-unit prostheses, or orthodontic bands or appliances. Sometimes cements are combined, as with reinforced zinc oxide eugenol cement and glass ionomer cement.

The term **luting** may be used instead of cementing. Dental cements are either temporary or permanent; they may also be used as a thermal base under a restoration.

■ ZINC PHOSPHATE CEMENT

Zinc phosphate is one of the oldest cements used in dentistry. This cement has a low solubility which resists breakdown in the mouth. Low thermoconductivity provides less sensitivity to hot and cold, and a long shelf life provides cost-effectiveness. Because of its history, zinc phosphate represents a standard by which current systems are measured.

Use

Zinc phosphate is used for permanent cementation of crowns, inlays, onlays, bridges, and orthodontic bands and brackets. It is also used as an insulating base under amalgam restorations. Zinc phosphate cement is supplied in a powder and a liquid and is always mixed on a glass slab (rather than on a paper mixing pad) (Figure 3-1).

Zinc oxide cement is dispensed and mixed differently, depending upon whether it is to

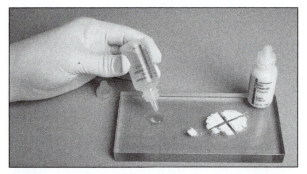

Figure 3-1 Zinc phosphate powder and liquid are dispensed onto a cool, dry glass slab. The powder is divided into increments; the liquid is dispensed by drops.

be used for permanent cementation or as an insulating base. (Both methods are described in the Practice Makes Perfect Procedure.)

Composition

Zinc oxide powder is comprised of zinc oxide and a small amount of magnesium oxide. It is available in a range of tooth-matching shades, having small amounts of pigment added to the powder.

The liquid, supplied in a bottle with an eyedropper–type stopper, is a solution of phosphoric acid and water buffered with agents to retard the setting time.

Zinc oxide cement liquid is acidic and therefore is irritating to the pulp; thus, the teeth must be protected with a base or liner prior to applying the cement.

When working with zinc oxide cement, one of the most important factors the dental

---

PRACTICE MAKES PERFECT PROCEDURE ▪ 3-1

Mixing Zinc Phosphate Cement (Powder and Liquid)

ARMAMENTARIUM
- Basic set-up
- Zinc phosphate powder
- Zinc phosphate liquid
- Cool, dry glass mixing slab
- Metal spatula
- Dappen dish
- Paper towels
- Sodium bicarbonate solution
- 2 × 2 gauze squares

PROCEDURE
1. Place the clean metal spatula and the cooled glass slab on a paper towel. Set out the bottles of zinc phosphate powder and liquid. [The glass slab is cooled by running it under cold water for several minutes or can be stored in the refrigerator, wrapped in a paper towel. It should be approximately 65–75°F (18–24°C).] When selecting the appropriate powder and liquid, the dental assistant should check to ensure that they are from the same manufacturer. (Never attempt to mix different manufacturers' products!)

2. Gently shake or fluff the bottle of powder before removing the cap.
3. To dispense the powder (Figure 3-2), squeeze out a small amount of powder onto the glass slab. [An amount approximately the size of a dime is sufficient for cementation of each unit (tooth) for which the cement is required.] Use the working end of the spatula, parallel to top of the glass slab, to flatten out the powder. Replace the bottle cap immediately to prevent accidental contamination or spillage.
4. Use the spatula to divide the powder into increments (Figure 3-3) as follows: Holding the spatula at a 90° angle to the glass slab, divide the zinc phosphate powder into two equal halves; divide each of these into quarters, then the first eight into sixteenths, and the last remaining quarter into eighths.
5. Swirl the liquid by gently shaking the bottle prior to dispensing. Dispense liquid from the dropper bottle according to the powder ratio required for the mixture (Figure 3-4). To produce uniform drops, hold the bottle vertically while dispensing the required number of drops.

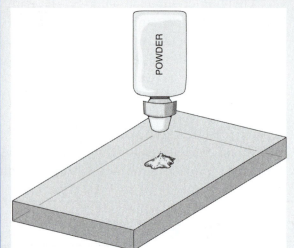

Figure 3-2 The dental assistant dispenses the zinc phosphate powder onto the glass slab.

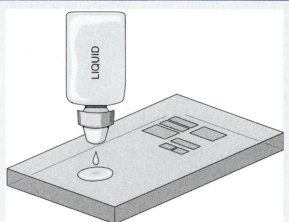

Figure 3-4 The dental assistant dispenses the liquid for zinc phosphate cement.

6. Place the correct number of drops (two for a base or eight for permanent cementation) onto the glass slab, approximately $1\frac{1}{2}$–2 inches from the powder.
7. Immediately replace the cap.
8. Grip the cement spatula with an overhand, with the index finger resting near the neck of the spatula blade and the thumb along the side of the spatula handle (see Figure 3-3).
9. Incorporate the first $\frac{1}{16}$ of the powder into the liquid. Use the flat side of the spatula blade to wet the powder particles.

10. Hold the spatula blade flat against the glass slab (Figure 3-5). Use a wide sweeping motion to spatulate the powder and liquid over a large area on the glass slab (Figure 3-6). Spatulate the first increment (small portion) of the powder for 15 seconds. Adding small amounts of powder helps neutralize the acid and achieves a smooth consistency. Each increment of powder must be thoroughly incorporated into the mix, with no unmixed particles of powder or liquid remaining on the spatula or around the outer edge of the mix.
11. Add the second increment, spatulate for 15 seconds; add the third increment and spatulate for 25 seconds.
12. Turn the spatula blade on edge and gather the mass with two or three strokes to check the consistency.

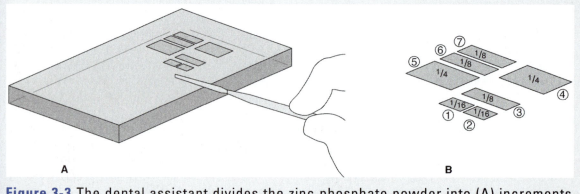

Figure 3-3 The dental assistant divides the zinc phosphate powder into (A) increments and (B) fractional portions.

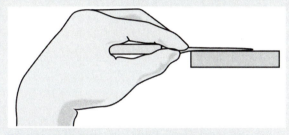

Figure 3-5 The dental assistant holds the cement spatula blade flat against the glass slab.

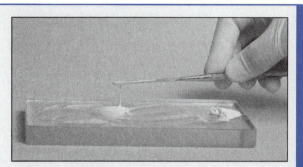

Figure 3-7 The 1-inch snap test indicates the zinc phosphate cement is ready for permanent cementation.

Repeat periodically during the incorporation of additional powder.

13. Continue adding larger increments into the mix until the desired consistency is reached within the prescribed time. The approximate time for each increment is 15, 15, 15, 20, 20, 15, and 20 seconds for a total spatulation time of 120 seconds (2 minutes).

14. Use the spatula to gather the entire mass into one unit on the glass slab. The consistency for permanent cementation is creamy and will follow the spatula for about 1 inch as it is tapped and lifted off the glass with the flat blade of the spatula before breaking into a thin thread. This is called the "1-inch snap test" (Figure 3-7). The cement is now ready to be loaded into the crown, bridge, inlay, or onlay, or into individual orthodontic bands upon the direction of the dentist. If the zinc phosphate is to be used as a thermal base, the consistency should be thick and puttylike (Figure 3-8).

15. Use the spatula to pick up the zinc phosphate and use your gloved fingers to roll the mass into a ball and either place it on the edge of the glass slab by "scraping" it onto the side of the slab and transferring the glass slab near the patient's chin and passing a placement instrument to the dentist or place the mass directly onto a plastic instrument and hand it to the dentist to be applied directly into the cavity preparation.

16. Use the 2×2 gauze sponge soaked in the sodium bicarbonate solution (in a dappen dish) to wipe the spatula clean, immediately after the cement is used. To further aid in clean-up, open up the 2×2 gauze soaked in sodium bicarbonate solution and place it over the slab to keep it soaked until clean-up, after the patient has been dismissed. This wiping and soaking prevents caking and hardening of the cement on the metal spatula and glass slab. (Dried zinc phosphate cement is very difficult to remove manually.)

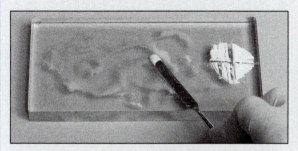

Figure 3-6 The dental assistant holds the cement spatula blade flat against the glass slab and incorporates the powder into the liquid, mixing over a large area to dissipate the heat released.

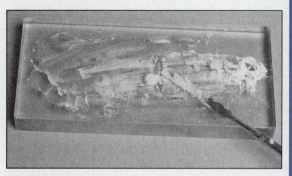

Figure 3-8 For use as a thermal base, zinc phosphate cement is of puttylike consistency and is incorporated into a ball.

assistant must keep in mind is that an **exothermic reaction** occurs. This means that heat is released, which accelerates the setting time of the cement. It may also irritate the pulp. The exothermic reaction requires that zinc oxide cement be mixed on a cool, dry glass slab over a wide area (never on a paper mixing pad).

Properties

When spatulated, zinc phosphate cement is high in strength, reaching two-thirds of its overall strength in less than 1 hour. Zinc phosphate sets within 5–9 minutes and has an extended mixing time of up to 2 minutes.

Mixing/Manipulation

The powder is dispensed onto the glass slab. Before dispensing it, the dental assistant should fluff the bottle. The liquid is dispensed by drops, onto the glass slab, near to but not touching the powder. Because the water content of the liquid is carefully established by the manufacturer, it must be maintained. Thus, when dispensing the liquid, the dental assistant should not leave the cap off; nor should the liquid be dispensed onto the mixing slab for a long time prior to use. Changes in humidity could affect the setting time and properties of the zinc phosphate cement.

The dental assistant must keep three factors in mind when preparing to mix and manipulate zinc phosphate cement. To slow the exothermic reaction and to help dissipate the resulting heat during spatulation:

1. Use a cool, dry glass slab (never paper).
2. Spread the mix over a large area of the glass slab when spatulating to increase working time.
3. Gradually add small increments (portions) of the powder to the liquid.

Of all the cements used in dentistry, zinc phosphate is the most critical. A thicker mix will set faster than a thin mix containing less powder.

■ ZINC OXIDE EUGENOL CEMENT

Zinc oxide eugenol (ZOE) cement is supplied in several forms: as a powder and a liquid, a two-paste system, capsules (mixed with an amalgamator), and syringes or capsules and in an automatrix system (Figure 3-9). Zinc oxide and eugenol have been used in dentistry for many years. There are two types of ZOE, which differ in their properties and uses.

Type I ZOE is less strong and is used for temporary restorations and for temporary

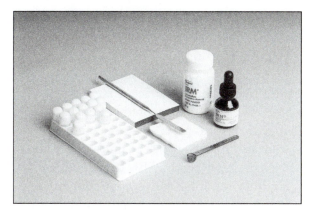

Figure 3-9 Intermediate ZOE is supplied in powder and liquid or capsule form.

cementation. Type II ZOE is reinforced and is stronger than type I. It is referred to as an intermediate restorative. Type II ZOE can last for 6–12 months. It is used when a tooth cannot be restored immediately (an example is when decay is very near to the pulp and must be allowed time to heal, pending a pulpotomy or root canal), when the patient has an extended illness, or when the patient is involved in an employment-related or military transfer.

Use

The special benefit of ZOE is that it has a sedative or soothing effect on the dental pulp. It is used as a temporary cement (Type I) or as an intermediate cement (Type II).

Composition

Type I zinc oxide powder contains zinc oxide, resin, zinc acetate, and an accelerator. The eugenol liquid contains oil of cloves (which is responsible for the characteristically familiar "dental office smell").

Type II reinforced zinc oxide powder also contains alumina and polymers (resins); the eugenol liquid contains ethoxybenzoic acid

(EBA). Noneugenol zinc oxide cements are available for patients who may experience sensitivity to eugenol.

Properties

Zinc oxide eugenol cement is very soluble in the mouth and thus dissolves fairly quickly. Reinforced ZOE has strength needed for permanent cementation and retention; however, it is not as strong as zinc phosphate cement and cannot be used indefinitely, as a permanent cement or restoration.

Zinc oxide eugenol cement has a neutral pH; because of its nonacidity and soothing effect on the pulp, a protective or insulating base or liner is not required with it.

Zinc oxide eugenol materials are not used under composite or acrylic restoration because eugenol is incompatible with these materials and also retards their setting process.

Mixing/Manipulation

Most often, ZOE cement is mixed with a metal spatula on a specially manufactured (coated) parchment mixing pad. This is to save clean-up time and to prevent the eugenol from soaking through the pad; in some instances, however, ZOE may be mixed on a glass slab to control or extend mixing time.

If the doctor prefers ZOE to be mixed on a glass slab, either different glass slabs must be used and identified as such or, if only one glass slab is used in the office, one side must be used for zinc phosphate cement only and the other must be used for ZOE only. This is to prevent an adverse reaction or a contaminated mix. Likewise, paper mixing pads supplied by the manufacturer should only be used for that specific type of cement and should not be interused, for the same reason—to prevent inadvertent contamination!

The dental assistant gently shakes the bottle of zinc oxide powder to agitate or fluff it; the assistant should gently swirl the eugenol liquid. The manufacturer supplies a powder dispenser and liquid dropper to use when dispensing ZOE.

The type and intended use of the material determine whether the powder is incorporated into the liquid in increments or all at once. The mixing time is usually 30–60 seconds.

All of the powder is incorporated into the liquid to form a uniform, smooth, creamy mix. Zinc oxide eugenol cement must be placed in the oral cavity fairly quickly because it is sensitive to moisture (saliva) and warmth.

If the ZOE cement is supplied in a two-paste system, one is the accelerator and one is a base. The two are dispensed in equal amounts (lengths) onto a paper mixing pad. The two pastes are mixed until a uniform color is achieved, usually within 10–15 seconds.

Setting time for ZOE is approximately 3–5 minutes. If used for temporary cementation,

PRACTICE MAKES PERFECT PROCEDURE ■ 3-2

Mixing Zinc Oxide Eugenol Cement (Powder and Liquid)

ARMAMENTARIUM
- Basic set-up
- Zinc oxide powder
- Eugenol
- Metal spatula
- Parchment mixing pad
- Measuring device
- Paper towels
- 91% alcohol or 70% ethyl alcohol
- 2 × 2 gauze squares

PROCEDURE
1. Fluff powder bottle before removing cap.
2. Dispense one scoop of powder from the large well of the measuring device and place on mixing pad. (A clean cement spatula may be used to dispense a portion of powder if one is not available.)
3. Replace the cap on the zinc oxide powder bottle to avoid accidental contamination or spillage.
4. Divide the zinc oxide powder into four equal portions.

5. Gently swirl the eugenol liquid bottle. Use the eyedropper to draw liquid from the bottle and hold the eyedropper perpendicularly (vertically) to the mixing pad.
6. Dispense one drop of eugenol liquid onto the parchment pad, above the powder but not touching it (Figure 3-10).
7. To spatulate the cement, using the flat part of the spatula blade, draw the first portion of the powder into the liquid and thoroughly spatulate; even pressure is required to wet all the particles of the powder. As the mixture becomes thicker, greater pressure may be required. Take care not to mix too vigorously, which may tear the parchment paper.
8. Next, draw the second portion of the zinc oxide powder into the mix and continue to spatulate. Repeat this procedure until the desired consistency is achieved. The consistency for temporary cementation of a crown or bridge is creamy (Figure 3-11) or puttylike for a base (Figure 3-12). It should be thick

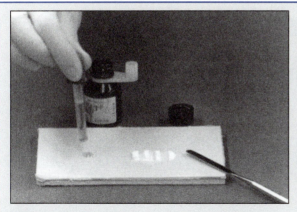

Figure 3-10 The dental assistant dispenses eugenol liquid onto the parchment mixing pad.

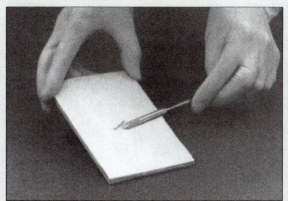

Figure 3-12 This is the puttylike consistency used for a ZOE base.

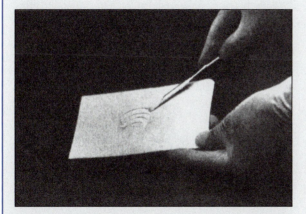

Figure 3-11 This is the creamy consistency desired for temporary cementation using ZOE.

enough to roll into a ball or cylinder with the blade of the spatula.

9. Next, bring the mixing pad and plastic placement instrument near to the patient's chin and pass the instrument to the dentist.

10. As soon as the dentist has finished using the cement, wipe the spatula and plastic placement instrument with a 2 × 2 gauze sponge dipped in alcohol.

11. To remove the top sheet of the parchment mixing pad, gently slide the clean spatula under the top sheet and discard it.

Special Considerations

- Always wipe the metal spatula and plastic instrument as the cement has been used to make clean-up easier.
- Always wear PPE when working at chairside.
- Maintain and work in a clean, dry, aseptic field.
- Clean and disinfect the work area at the conclusion of the procedure, after dismissing the patient.
- Always follow OSHA regulations and CDC recommendations to help prevent the spread of bloodborne diseases and to protect dental personnel.

Mixing Zinc Oxide Eugenol Cement (Two-Paste System)

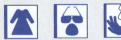

ARMAMENTARIUM

- Basic set-up
- Two-paste zinc oxide eugenol system (accelerator and base)
- Paper mixing pad
- Cement spatula
- 2 × 2 gauze sponges (moistened)
- 91% alcohol or 70% ethyl alcohol
- Plastic instrument

PROCEDURE

1. Dispense equal amounts of the material required for the procedure as directed by the dentist. Extrude (squeeze out) of the respective tubes, parallel to and close to each other, but not touching until mixing time. Replace caps immediately.

2. Use the edge of the blade to pick up one of the ribbons of paste and mix it into the other into a homogenous mass, mixing over a small area. Spread the mix over a small area, then gather; repeat. The ZOE material should be creamy.

3. Use the 2 × 2 gauze to wipe both sides of the spatula clean; gather all the material into one area to load into the prosthesis, as indicated. Either load the prosthesis under the dentist's direction or pass it to the dentist, holding the parchment mixing pad near the patient's chin, and pass the plastic instrument to the dentist.

4. After the prosthesis has been successfully loaded with ZOE, use another alcohol-moistened 2 × 2 gauze sponge to wipe the excess ZOE from the spatula and plastic instrument to prevent caking and hardening (which is harder to remove later).

Special Considerations

- Always wipe the metal spatula and plastic instrument as the cement has been used to make clean-up easier.
- Always wear PPE when working at chairside.
- Maintain and work in a clean, dry, aseptic field.
- Clean and disinfect the work area at the conclusion of the procedure, after dismissing the patient.
- Always follow OSHA regulations and CDC recommendations to help prevent the spread of bloodborne diseases and to protect dental personnel.

the consistency is smooth and creamy; if used as a temporary restoration, it should be of puttylike consistency.

■ POLYCARBOXYLATE CEMENT

Polycarboxylate cement (sometimes referred to as **zinc polyacrylate cement**) is a permanent cement also used as an insulating base. It is supplied as a powder and a viscous liquid and is the first dental cement with the ability to chemically bond to the tooth structure.

Use

Polycarboxylate cement is used for permanent cementation of crowns, bridges, inlays, and onlays; for orthodontic bands, brackets, and appliances; as an insulating base; and as a temporary restoration.

Composition

Polycarboxylate cement powder is similar to zinc phosphate with zinc oxide as the main component; it may also contain a small amount of magnesium oxide. Some manufacturers substitute magnesium oxide with stannous fluoride, which increases strength and reduces film thickness. It is supplied in a bottle with a dispenser (pipette). The liquid is a viscous solution of polyacrylic acid and water. It is supplied in a squeeze bottle or in calibrated syringes. Self-adhesive resin cements are also available that do not involve a bottle and syringes, thereby eliminating etching, priming, and handling steps (Figure 3-13).

Properties

Polycarboxylate cement sets in 3–5 minutes and does not produce an exothermic reaction;

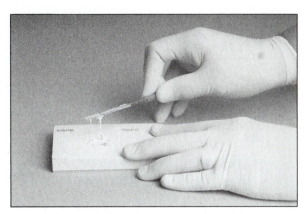

Figure 3-13 RelyX Unicem self-adhesive universal resin cement.
(Courtesy of 3M ESPE.)

it is therefore considered to be "kind" to the pulp. It bonds chemically to tooth structure and mechanically to restorations. Its strength is similar to that of reinforced ZOE and less than that of zinc phosphate cement. Although polycarboxylate cement has a more viscous consistency, it flows readily when applied to a surface. Because the liquid contains water, polycarboxylate cement has a shelf life. Should the liquid become discolored, it should be discarded.

When the powder and liquid are mixed together, the result is an extremely high acid at the time of placement, a pH of 1.7. The acid is rapidly neutralized, however, during the setting time.

Mixing/Manipulation

Polycarboxylate cement can be mixed on either a glass or a paper mixing pad using a metal spatula. The powder is fluffed prior to dispensing. The viscous liquid is dispensed from a squeeze bottle or a calibrated syringe. The dental assistant holds the squeeze bottle perpendicularly to the mixing pad or glass slab and squeezes it until one drop falls next to but not touching the powder.

Mixing Polycarboxylate Cement

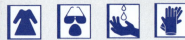

ARMAMENTARIUM

- Basic set-up
- Polycarboxylate cement powder
- Polycarboxylate liquid squeeze or calibrated syringe dispenser
- Nonabsorbent paper mixing pad (or a glass slab)
- Polycarboxylate cement powder measuring scoop
- Cement spatula
- 2 × 2 gauze sponges (moistened with a 10% sodium hydroxide solution)
- Minute timer
- Plastic instrument

PROCEDURE

1. Fluff the polycarboxylate powder; dispense using the scoop provided by the manufacturer. Dispense one scoop of powder onto the mixing pad or glass slab by pressing the measuring scoop firmly into the powder. Withdraw the scoop from the bottle, removing excess powder with the cement spatula. The powder should be flush with the top of the measuring scoop. Replace the bottle cap to prevent accidental contamination or spillage.

2. Extrude three drops of liquid on the mixing pad, near to but not touching the powder. (Liquid should not be placed on the mixing pad or glass slab until just prior to mixing because exposure to air may cause loss of water, resulting in the premature thickening of the mix.) If the liquid is dispensed from a plastic squeeze bottle, hold the bottle vertically and squeeze. Release pressure when the drop separates fully from the nozzle tip. If a calibrated liquid dispenser is being used, press the plunger rod to release three full calibrations as indicated on the plunger barrel.

3. Mixing quickly, in a folding motion while applying moderate pressure, incorporate the powder into the liquid in one increment. Spatulation should be completed within 30 seconds. (A timer is helpful when practicing the procedure.) Do not overspatulate.

4. The consistency of polycarboxylate cement for permanent cementation is smooth and creamy and the mass will flow from the spatula in a thin strand. The mix will be slightly more viscous than zinc phosphate cement. The cement must be applied to the tooth and the object to be cemented while the mix is glossy. Gather the cement into a mass, wiping both sides of the spatula. Should the cement lose its sheen or become stringy, do not use it because it has already begun to set. Start over with a fresh mix on a clean mixing pad with a clean spatula.

5. For a base, less liquid should be used, according to the manufacturer's instructions. The consistency should also be glossy; however, the consistency should be tacky and stiff. To facilitate or accelerate the setting of the base, dip the plastic placement instrument in excess powder or in alcohol. Setting time is 3–5 minutes.

6. If the polycarboxylate cement is to be applied directly to the tooth (whether as a permanent cement or an insulating base), mass the mixture together and bring it near to the patient's chin and pass a plastic instrument to the dentist for application.

7. Clean-up should be done immediately after placing the cement to avoid caking and hardening of the cement, which is much more difficult to remove later. Wipe the spatula with a wet 2 × 2 gauze sponge soaked in a 10 percent sodium hydroxide solution. To remove the top sheet of the mixing pad, place the cleaned spatula flat underneath the top sheet and tear it off. Fold and discard the used paper mixing sheet to prevent accidental sticking or contamination of other items on the instrument tray set-up.

Special Considerations

- Always wipe the metal spatula and plastic instrument as the cement has been used to make clean-up easier.
- Always wear PPE when working at chairside.
- Maintain and work in a clean, dry, aseptic field.
- Clean and disinfect the work area at the conclusion of the procedure, after dismissing the patient.
- Always follow OSHA regulations and CDC recommendations to help prevent the spread of bloodborne diseases and to protect dental personnel.

Spatulation is completed in 30–60 seconds; the working time is 3 minutes. If the mixed cement takes on a stringy consistency or a shiny or cobwebbed appearance, it is over-spatulated and should not be used. It should be discarded and a new mix should be started.

Prior to cementing an orthodontic appliance or crown or fixed bridge, the dentist may choose to acid etch the tooth surface. This helps strengthen the bond between the tooth surface and the appliance or prosthesis being cemented.

If used for cementing gold or porcelain restorations, the restoration must be thoroughly cleansed prior to cementation. This is to remove contaminants, such as chemical residue remaining from the acid pickling solution, which, if allowed to remain, prevents the cement from adhering to the restoration. The underside of the gold restoration should be cleaned with an air abrasive or an abrasive burr and then washed and thoroughly dried.

■ GLASS IONOMER CEMENT

Glass ionomer cement is a new cementation system with a variety of applications in dentistry. It is supplied as a powder and liquid, paste systems, and syringes and in capsule forms. Glass ionomers are also supplied in either self-curing or light-curing systems.

Use

Type I glass ionomer is a finer grain glass ionomer and is used for permanent cementation of crowns and bridges and for orthodontic bonding; it may also be used for pit and fissure sealants, which are addressed in Chapter 9.

Type II glass ionomer is coarser and is supplied in a variety of shades to match tooth color. It is used in Class III and V permanent restorations, addressed in Chapter 4.

Type III glass ionomer is used as a liner and dentin bonding agent (dentin replacement or base material).

Type IV glass ionomer is used for crown and core buildups.

Composition

Glass ionomer powder is a silicate glass powder containing calcium, aluminum, and fluoride (calcium fluoroaluminosilicate glass). The liquid is an aqueous solution of polyacrylic acid. Glass ionomer cement is available as a powder and liquid system and in capsules. The capsules require a high-speed amalgamator to mix the cement.

Properties

Glass ionomer cement is strong enough to be a supportive base and is similar to zinc phosphate cement in strength. It mechanically and chemically bonds to tooth structures. Glass ionomer releases fluoride, which prevents secondary decay by strengthening tooth structure.

Glass ionomers are nonirritating; complete setting time takes up to 24 hours.

Mixing/Manipulation

Glass ionomer cements can be mixed on either a paper mixing pad or a cool glass slab. A paper mixing pad is desirable because of ease and speed of clean-up; however, a cooled glass slab may be used to retard working and/or setting time.

If the practice uses more than one type of cement that is mixed on a glass slab, different slabs must be used; if only one glass slab is used, sides must be marked according to the type of cement being mixed on either side. To avoid cross-contamination, sides or slabs should not be interused.

The cement is mixed quickly, according to the manufacturer's instructions; due to the water content of the liquid, which may evaporate, the liquid should not be dispensed until prior to use.

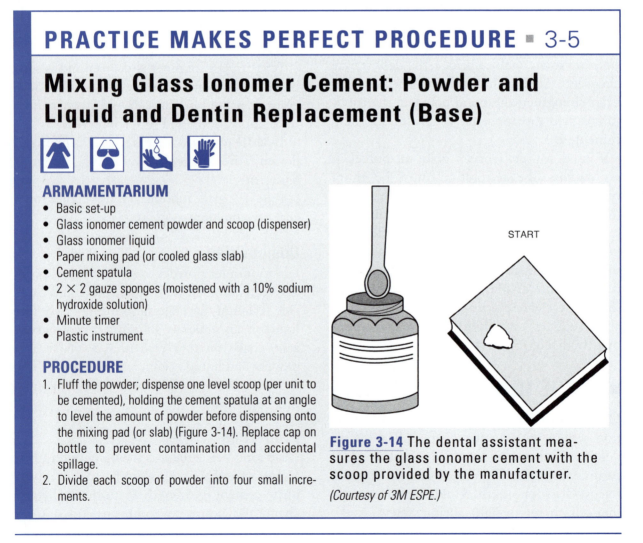

PRACTICE MAKES PERFECT PROCEDURE ▪ 3-5

Mixing Glass Ionomer Cement: Powder and Liquid and Dentin Replacement (Base)

ARMAMENTARIUM
- Basic set-up
- Glass ionomer cement powder and scoop (dispenser)
- Glass ionomer liquid
- Paper mixing pad (or cooled glass slab)
- Cement spatula
- 2 × 2 gauze sponges (moistened with a 10% sodium hydroxide solution)
- Minute timer
- Plastic instrument

PROCEDURE
1. Fluff the powder; dispense one level scoop (per unit to be cemented), holding the cement spatula at an angle to level the amount of powder before dispensing onto the mixing pad (or slab) (Figure 3-14). Replace cap on bottle to prevent contamination and accidental spillage.
2. Divide each scoop of powder into four small increments.

Figure 3-14 The dental assistant measures the glass ionomer cement with the scoop provided by the manufacturer.
(Courtesy of 3M ESPE.)

3. Holding the liquid bottle vertically, squeeze and dispense two drops of liquid, per unit to be cemented, onto the mixing pad (Figure 3-15) just prior to spatulation. (Always keep bottles tightly sealed when not in use.)

4. Using the spatula at an angle, draw the first increment of powder into the liquid, mixing over a small area. With the flat blade of the spatula mix each increment thoroughly before adding the next increment (Figure 3-16). Spatulation should be completed within 60 seconds. Glass ionomer cement should have a glossy appearance. If extended working time is desired, as when cementing individual multiple units, a cooled, dry glass slab or multiple mixes work well.

As a Dentin Replacement (Base)

1. Select the desired shade of powder to match the dentin shade.

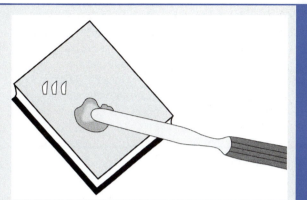

Figure 3-16 The dental assistant adds increments of powder, incorporating the powder into the liquid.

(Courtesy of 3M ESPE.)

2. Dispense one level scoop of powder onto the mixing pad and divide into small increments.

3. Hold the liquid vertically and dispense one drop of liquid onto the mixing pad.

4. Draw the first increment of powder into the liquid. Spatulate each increment thoroughly before adding the next. Complete spatulation within 30 seconds. The consistency should be puttylike and tacky.

5. Bring the thoroughly mixed cement into a mass and wipe the spatula clean with a moist 2 × 2 gauze sponge. Bring the mixing pad or slab close to the patient's chin and pass the plastic placement instrument to the dentist.

6. When the dentist has finished applying the glass ionomer cement, use another 2 × 2 gauze sponge to remove any remaining cement from the plastic instrument, spatula, or glass slab. To clean up, remove the top paper layer of the mixing pad by "slicing" around the edge(s) of the pad, holding the spatula in a horizontal position. Fold the paper prior to disposal to prevent inadvertent spillage or contamination of the instrument tray.

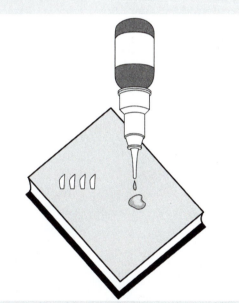

Figure 3-15 The dental assistant dispenses glass ionomer liquid onto the mixing pad.

(Courtesy of 3M ESPE.)

Special Considerations

- Always wipe the metal spatula and plastic instrument as the cement has been used to make clean-up easier.
- Always wear PPE when working at chairside.
- Maintain and work in a clean, dry, aseptic field.
- Clean and disinfect the work area at the conclusion of the procedure, after dismissing the patient.
- Always follow OSHA regulations and CDC recommendations to help prevent the spread of bloodborne diseases and to protect dental personnel.

PRACTICE MAKES PERFECT PROCEDURE ▪ 3-6

Mixing Glass Ionomer Cement: Using an Amalgamator

ARMAMENTARIUM
- Basic set-up
- High-speed amalgamator
- Glass ionomer capsule activator
- Glass ionomer powder and liquid capsule

PROCEDURE
1. Activate the glass ionomer cement capsule with the activator supplied by the manufacturer (Figure 3-17).
2. Insert the activated capsule into the high-speed amalgamator.
3. Triturate (mix) the activated capsule for 10 seconds.
4. Remove the capsule, insert into the applicator, and immediately remove the sealing pin. Position the nozzle tip of the capsule at 90° to the cavity preparation for optimal access to the cavity preparation.
5. Pass the applicator to the dentist, handle first, for the cement to be expressed directly into the tooth preparation by squeezing. Working time is from $1\frac{1}{2}$ to 2 minutes.

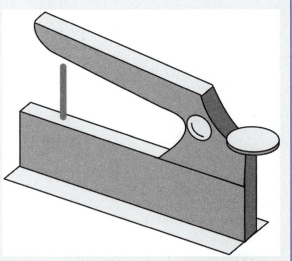

Figure 3-17 The dental assistant activates the glass ionomer cement capsule with the activator supplied by the manufacturer.

(Courtesy of 3M ESPE.)

While having many of the properties of polycarboxylate cement, the liquid of glass ionomer cement is not as viscous and is therefore easier to dispense and spatulate.

The powder is fluffed prior to dispensing, then measured out using the scoop (dispenser) supplied by the manufacturer. Then the liquid is dispensed prior to spatulation. Mixing time is 30–60 seconds. Setting time is approximately 5 minutes.

■ CRITICAL THINKING QUESTIONS

1. Why is it important to use a cool, dry glass slab when mixing zinc phosphate cement?

2. Why is a specially treated parchment paper pad used to mix ZOE?

3. Why should polycarboxylate cement liquid not be dispensed until just prior to use?

4. When either a paper or cooled glass slab may be used for mixing cement, why is a paper mixing pad preferable? When is a glass slab preferable?

5. When the dentist prefers more than one type of cement used in the office to be mixed on a glass slab, why must different slabs be used OR, if there is only one slab, why must each side be marked for use of the respective slab?

PRACTICE MAKES PERFECT
STUDENT ASSESSMENT 3-1

Mixing Zinc Phosphate Cement (Powder and Liquid)

Student's Name: _____

Date: _____   Instructor: _____

Note: The blank space is provided for the instructor to check off the student's progress. The student may practice the procedure as many times as necessary before being evaluated. Some portions of the exercise may be performed on a typodont, stone tooth model, or extracted tooth or simulated in a clinical operatory. The student has successfully completed the following:

_____ Worn necessary PPE

_____ Assembled necessary armamentarium

_____ Maintained a clear, dry, aseptic working field

_____ Placed the clean metal spatula and the cooled glass slab on a paper towel

_____ Set out the bottles of zinc phosphate powder and liquid

_____ Fluffed powder bottle before removing cap

_____ Dispensed the powder onto the glass slab, approximately the size of a dime, for each unit (tooth) for which the cement is required

_____ Used the working end of the spatula, parallel to top of the glass slab, to flatten the powder

_____ Replaced the bottle cap immediately to prevent accidental contamination or spillage

_____ Used the flat blade of the spatula to flatten the powder

_____ Held the spatula at a 90° angle to the glass slab to divide the zinc phosphate powder into increments as directed

_____ Swirled the liquid by gently shaking the bottle prior to dispensing

_____ Dispensed liquid from the dropper bottle according to the powder ratio required for the mixture, producing uniform drops

_____ Placed the correct number of drops (two for a base or eight for permanent cementation) onto the glass slab, approximately $1\frac{1}{2}$–2 inches from the powder

_____ Replaced the cap immediately

_____ Gripped the cement spatula with an overhand, with the index finger resting near the neck of the spatula blade and the thumb along the side of the spatula handle

_____ Incorporated the first $\frac{1}{16}$ of the powder into the liquid using the flat side of the spatula blade to wet the powder particles

_____ Held the spatula flat and used a wide sweeping motion to spatulate the powder and liquid over a large area on the glass slab

_____ Spatulated the first increment (small portion) of the powder for 15 seconds and added small amounts of powder to achieve a smooth consistency

_____ Added the second increment and spatulated for 15 seconds

_____ Added the third increment and spatulated for 25 seconds

_____ Turned the spatula blade on edge and gathered the mass with two or three strokes to check the consistency

_____ Repeated this step periodically during the incorporation of additional powder

_____ Continued to add larger increments into the mix until the desired consistency was reached within the prescribed time [The approximate time for each increment was 15, 15, 15, 20, 20, 15, and 20 seconds, for a total spatulation time of 120 seconds (2 minutes).]

_____ Used the spatula to gather the entire mass into one unit on the glass slab. The consistency for permanent cementation was creamy and followed the spatula for about 1 inch as it was tapped and lifted off the glass with the flat blade of the spatula before breaking into a thin thread. (This is called the 1-inch snap test.)

_____ Used the spatula to pick up the zinc phosphate and gloved fingers to roll the mass into a ball; then either placed it on the edge of the glass slab by "scraping" it onto the side of the slab and transferring the glass slab near to the patient's chin and passing a placement instrument to the dentist; or placed the mass directly onto a plastic instrument and handed it to the dentist to be applied directly into the cavity preparation (If the zinc phosphate was to be used as a thermal base, the consistency was thick and puttylike.)

_____ Used the 2 × 2 gauze sponge soaked in sodium bicarbonate solution (in a dappen dish) to wipe the spatula clean, immediately after the cement was used

_____ Opened up the 2 × 2 gauze soaked in sodium bicarbonate solution and placed it over the slab to keep it soaked until clean-up, after the patient was dismissed

_____ Cleaned and disinfected the work area at the conclusion of the procedure, after dismissing the patient

_____ Followed OSHA regulations and CDC recommendations to help prevent the spread of bloodborne diseases and to protect dental personnel

Comments

_____
_____
_____
_____
_____

PRACTICE MAKES PERFECT
STUDENT ASSESSMENT 3-2

Mixing Zinc Oxide Eugenol Cement (Powder and Liquid)

Student's Name: _____

Date: _____   Instructor: _____

Note: The blank space is provided for the instructor to check off the student's progress. The student may practice the procedure as many times as necessary before being evaluated. Some portions of the exercise may be performed on a typodont, stone tooth model, or extracted tooth or simulated in a clinical operatory. The student has successfully completed the following:

_____ Worn necessary PPE

_____ Assembled necessary armamentarium

_____ Maintained a clear, dry, aseptic working field

_____ Fluffed powder bottle before removing cap

_____ Dispensed one scoop of powder from the large well of the measuring device and placed on mixing pad

_____ Replaced the cap on the zinc oxide powder bottle

_____ Divided the zinc oxide powder into four equal portions

_____ Gently swirled the eugenol liquid bottle

_____ Used the eyedropper to dispense one drop of eugenol liquid onto the treated parchment pad, near the powder but not touching it

_____ Spatulated the cement, using the flat part of the spatula blade, to draw the first portion of the powder into the liquid and thoroughly spatulated it, using even pressure to wet all the particles of the powder

_____ Drew the second portion of the zinc oxide powder into the mix and continued to spatulate

_____ Repeated this procedure until the desired consistency was achieved (The consistency for temporary cementation of a crown or bridge was creamy or putty-like for a base.)

_____ Brought the mixing pad and plastic placement instrument near to the patient's chin and passed the instrument to the dentist

_____ At the completion of the application wiped the spatula and plastic placement instrument with a 2 × 2 gauze sponge dipped in alcohol

_____ Removed the top sheet of the parchment mixing pad and gently slid the clean spatula under the top sheet and discarded it

_____ Cleaned and disinfected the work area at the conclusion of the procedure, after dismissing the patient

_____ Followed OSHA regulations and CDC recommendations to help prevent the spread of bloodborne diseases and to protect dental personnel

Comments

_____

_____

_____

_____

_____

PRACTICE MAKES PERFECT
STUDENT ASSESSMENT 3-3

Mixing Zinc Oxide Eugenol Cement (Two-Paste System)

Student's Name: _____

Date: _____   Instructor: _____

Note: The blank space is provided for the instructor to check off the student's progress. The student may practice the procedure as many times as necessary before being evaluated. Some portions of the exercise may be performed on a typodont, stone tooth model, or extracted tooth or simulated in a clinical operatory. The student has successfully completed the following:

_____ Worn necessary PPE

_____ Assembled necessary armamentarium

_____ Maintained a clear, dry, aseptic working field

_____ Dispensed equal amounts of the material required by extruding the material parallel to and close to each other but not touching until mixing time, and replaced caps immediately

_____ Used the edge of the blade to pick up one of the ribbons of paste and mixed it into the other to form a homogenous mass

_____ Spread the mix over a small area, then gathered and repeated, creating a creamy mixture

_____ Used the 2 × 2 gauze to wipe both sides of the spatula clean

_____ Gathered all of the material into one area to load into the prosthesis, as indicated

_____ Held the parchment mixing pad near the patient's chin and passed the plastic instrument to the dentist

_____ After the prosthesis was successfully loaded with ZOE, used another moistened 2 × 2 gauze sponge to wipe the excess ZOE from the spatula and plastic instrument to prevent caking and hardening

_____ Cleaned and disinfected the work area at the conclusion of the procedure, after dismissing the patient

_____ Followed OSHA regulations and CDC recommendations to help prevent the spread of bloodborne diseases and to protect dental personnel

Comments

_____

_____

_____

_____

_____

Mixing Polycarboxylate Cement

Student's Name: _____

Date: _____   Instructor: _____

Note: The blank space is provided for the instructor to check off the student's progress. The student may practice the procedure as many times as necessary before being evaluated. Some portions of the exercise may be performed on a typodont, stone tooth model, or extracted tooth or simulated in a clinical operatory. The student has successfully completed the following:

_____ Worn necessary PPE

_____ Assembled necessary armamentarium

_____ Maintained a clear, dry, aseptic working field

_____ Fluffed the polycarboxylate powder prior to dispensing with the scoop provided by the manufacturer

_____ Dispensed one scoop of powder onto the mixing pad or glass slab by pressing the measuring scoop firmly into the powder

_____ Withdrew the scoop from the bottle, removing excess powder with the edge of the cement spatula blade, making the powder flush with the top of the measuring scoop

_____ Replaced the bottle cap to prevent accidental contamination or spillage

_____ Extruded three drops of liquid on the mixing pad, near to but not touching the powder

_____ If the liquid was dispensed from a plastic squeeze bottle, held it vertically and squeezed, releasing pressure when the drops separated fully from the nozzle tip. If a calibrated liquid dispenser was used, the plunger rod was pressed to release three full calibrations as indicated on the plunger barrel.

_____ Mixed the cement quickly in a folding motion while applying moderate pressure and incorporated the powder into the liquid in one increment. Spatulation was completed within 30 seconds.

_____ Ensured the consistency of polycarboxylate cement for permanent cementation was smooth and creamy

_____ Ensured the consistency for a base was glossy but tacky and stiff

_____ Massed the mixture together and brought it near to the patient's chin and passed the plastic instrument to the dentist for application

_____ Immediately cleaned up to avoid caking and hardening of the cement by wiping the spatula with a wet 2 × 2 gauze sponge soaked in a 10 percent sodium hydroxide solution

_____ Cleaned and disinfected the work area at the conclusion of the procedure, after dismissing the patient

_____ Followed OSHA regulations and CDC recommendations to help prevent the spread of bloodborne diseases and to protect dental personnel

Comments

_____

_____

_____

_____

_____

Mixing Glass Ionomer Cement: Powder and Liquid and Dentin Replacement (Base)

Student's Name: _____

Date: _____   Instructor: _____

Note: The blank space is provided for the instructor to check off the student's progress. The student may practice the procedure as many times as necessary before being evaluated. Some portions of the exercise may be performed on a typodont, stone tooth model, or extracted tooth or simulated in a clinical operatory. The student has successfully completed the following:

_____ Worn necessary PPE

_____ Assembled necessary armamentarium

_____ Maintained a clear, dry, aseptic working field

_____ Fluffed the powder; dispensed one level scoop (per unit to be cemented), holding the cement spatula at an angle to level the amount of powder before dispensing onto the mixing pad (or slab)

_____ Replaced cap on bottle to prevent contamination and accidental spillage

_____ Divided each scoop of powder into four small increments

_____ Holding the liquid bottle vertically, squeezed and dispensed two drops of liquid, per unit to be cemented, onto the mixing pad just prior to spatulation

_____ Using the spatula at an angle, drew the first increment of powder into the liquid, mixing over a small area and, with the flat blade of the spatula, mixed each increment thoroughly before adding the next increment

_____ Completed spatulation within 60 seconds

As a Dentin Replacement (Base)

_____ Selected the desired shade of powder to match the dentin shade

_____ Dispensed one level scoop of powder onto the mixing pad and divided it into small increments

_____ Held the liquid vertically and dispensed one drop of liquid onto the mixing pad

_____ Drew the first increment of powder into the liquid

_____ Spatulated each increment thoroughly before adding the next

_____ Completed spatulation within 30 seconds; the consistency was puttylike and tacky

_____ Brought the thoroughly mixed cement into a mass and wiped the spatula clean with a moist 2 × 2 gauze sponge

_____ Brought the mixing pad or slab close to the patient's chin and passed the plastic placement instrument to the dentist

_____ When the dentist was finished applying the glass ionomer cement, used another 2 × 2 gauze sponge to remove any remaining cement from the plastic instrument, spatula, or glass slab

_____ Cleaned and disinfected the work area at the conclusion of the procedure, after dismissing the patient

_____ Followed OSHA regulations and CDC recommendations to help prevent the spread of bloodborne diseases and to protect dental personnel

Comments

_____

_____

_____

_____

_____

Mixing Glass Ionomer Cement: Using an Amalgamator

Student's Name: _____

Date: _____   Instructor: _____

Note: The blank space is provided for the instructor to check off the student's progress. The student may practice the procedure as many times as necessary before being evaluated. Some portions of the exercise may be performed on a typodont, stone tooth model, or extracted tooth or simulated in a clinical operatory. The student has successfully completed the following:

_____ Worn necessary PPE

_____ Assembled necessary armamentarium

_____ Maintained a clear, dry, aseptic working field

_____ Activated the glass ionomer cement capsule with the activator supplied by the manufacturer

_____ Inserted the activated capsule into the high-speed amalgamator

_____ Triturated the activated capsule for 10 seconds

_____ Removed the capsule, inserted it into the applicator, and immediately removed the sealing pin

_____ Positioned the nozzle tip of the capsule at 90° to the cavity preparation for optimal access to the cavity preparation

_____ Passed the applicator to the dentist, handle first, for the cement to be expressed directly into the tooth preparation by squeezing; working time was from $1\frac{1}{2}$ to 2 minutes

_____ Cleaned and disinfected the work area at the conclusion of the procedure, after dismissing the patient

_____ Followed OSHA regulations and CDC recommendations to help prevent the spread of bloodborne diseases and to protect dental personnel

Comments

_____
_____
_____
_____
_____

CHAPTER 3: POSTTEST

Instructions: For each of the following, select the answer that most accurately completes the question or statement.

1. All of the following are true about light-cured cements *except*
   A. They are usually hand mixed by the dental assistant.
   B. They are easier to work with.
   C. They give the operator additional manipulation and working time prior to initiating the final cure.

2. Dental cements are used
   A. alone or in combination with other dental materials
   B. to lute veneers
   C. to lute single-unit or multiple-unit prostheses
   D. to lute orthodontic bands or appliances
   E. for all of the above

3. Zinc phosphate cement is supplied in a powder and a liquid and is always mixed on a paper mixing pad.
   A. True
   B. False

4. All of the following are true of zinc oxide cement *except*
   A. The liquid is acidic and irritating to the pulp.
   B. Its use requires the tooth or teeth be protected with a base or liner prior to applying the cement.
   C. It is soothing to the pulp.
   D. It gives off an exothermic reaction when mixed.

5. When dispensing zinc phosphate liquid, the dental assistant should replace the cap immediately and should not dispense the liquid onto the mixing slab for a long time prior to use. This is because:
   A. Changes in humidity could affect setting time and properties of the zinc phosphate cement.
   B. The water content of the liquid is carefully established by the manufacturer and must be maintained.
   C. Leaving the cap off creates an exothermic reaction.
   D. A and B only
   E. B and C only

6. To slow the exothermic reaction and to help dissipate the resulting heat during spatulation of zinc phosphate cement, the dental assistant should
   A. use a cool, dry glass slab (never paper)
   B. spread the mix over a large area of the glass slab when spatulating to increase working time
   C. gradually add small increments of the powder to the liquid
   D. A and B only
   E. B and C only
   F. all of the above

7. When working with dental cements, the dental assistant can mix different manufacturers' products to save time and money on dental supplies.
   A. True
   B. False

8. When working with dental cement powder the dental assistant should replace the bottle cap immediately to do all of the following *except*
   A. prevent accidental contamination
   B. prevent spillage
   C. aerate the liquid
   D. A and B only
   E. B and C only

9. All of the following are true with regard to type II ZOE *except* it
   A. is weaker and thus is used only for temporary restorations and temporary cementation
   B. is reinforced and is stronger than type I
   C. is referred to as an intermediate restorative
   D. can last for 6–12 months
   E. is used when a tooth cannot be restored immediately due to close proximity to the dental pulp

10. Due to its neutral pH and soothing effect on the pulp, a protective or insulating base or liner is not required when applying zinc oxide eugenol cement.
    A. True
    B. False

11. Zinc oxide eugenol materials are not used under composite or acrylic restorations because eugenol
    A. is compatible with these materials
    B. is irritating to the pulp
    C. retards the setting process
    D. accelerates the setting process too quickly to allow sufficient working time for the operator

12. If the doctor prefers more than one cement to be mixed on a glass slab, either different glass slabs must be used and identified as such or, if only one glass slab is used in the office, each side must be used for mixing a specific cement only. Why?
    A. to save money on the purchase of multiple glass slabs
    B. to prevent an adverse reaction or a contaminated mix
    C. to prevent clutter caused by too many paper mixing pads
    D. all of the above

13. Zinc oxide eugenol cement must be placed in the oral cavity fairly quickly because
    A. of the resulting exothermic reaction
    B. contamination from using too much powder may result
    C. the dental assistant may be required to perform other duties in the office at the same time the cement is being placed
    D. it is sensitive to moisture (saliva) and warmth

14. Zinc oxide eugenol should be mixed over a _____ area until homogenous and creamy in appearance.
    A. small
    B. medium
    C. large
    D. very large

15. Polycarboxylate cement is used for all of the following applications *except*
    A. for permanent cementation of crowns, bridges, inlays, and onlays
    B. for orthodontic bands, brackets, and appliances
    C. as an insulating base
    D. as a temporary cement
    E. as a temporary restoration

16. All of the following are true with regard to polycarboxylate cement *except* it
    A. has a viscous consistency yet flows readily when applied to a surface
    B. sets in 3–5 minutes
    C. is kind to the pulp
    D. bonds chemically to tooth structure and mechanically to restorations
    E. produces an exothermic reaction

17. If mixed polycarboxylate cement takes on a stringy consistency or a shiny or cobwebbed appearance, it
    A. is overspatulated and should not be used
    B. should be discarded and a new mix should be begun
    C. is giving off an exothermic reaction and will quickly cool down
    D. A and B only
    E. all of the above

18. When mixed properly for permanent cementation, polycarboxylate cement should pass the 1-inch snap test.
    A. True
    B. False

19. Glass ionomer releases fluoride, which prevents secondary decay by strengthening tooth structure.
    A. True
    B. False

20. Mixing time for glass ionomer cement is _____ seconds.
    A. 12–15
    B. 15–30
    C. 30–60
    D. 60–120

Restorative Materials

Chapter 4 Restorative Dental Materials

To be a co-worker—creating a spirit of co-operation and friendliness rather than one of fault-finding and criticism.

To be enthusiastic—for therein lies the easiest way to accomplishment.

To be generous, not alone of my name but of my praise and my time.

Excerpt from the "Creed for Dental Assistants" by Juliette A. Southard.
Reprinted with the permission of the American Dental Assistants Association, Chicago, IL.

RESTORATIVE DENTAL MATERIALS · CHAPTER 4

LEARNING OBJECTIVES

Upon completion of this chapter the student should be able to:

1. Discuss the general types of restorative materials used in dentistry and their specific applications.

2. Describe the role and duties of the dental assistant in the use, instrumentation, manipulation, application, and clean-up procedures required when placing amalgam restorations.

3. Describe the role and duties of the dental assistant in safe handling of mercury, the principles of mercury hygiene, and the necessary steps required to safely clean up a mercury spill.

4. Describe the role and duties of the dental assistant in the use, instrumentation, manipulation, application, and clean-up procedures required when placing composite restorations.

5. Describe the role and duties of the dental assistant in the use, instrumentation, manipulation, application, and clean-up procedures required when placing glass ionomer restorations.

KEY TERMS

amalgam/amalgamator
composite
Material Safety Data
   Sheets (MSDSs)

trituration/triturator

INTRODUCTION

Chairside restorative (filling) materials represent many advancements in modern dentistry. At one time, surgery was often the only remedy available to alleviate tooth pain and to eradicate the ravages associated with dental caries. Today's restorative materials play a significant role in helping patients retain their natural dentition.

The most commonly used chairside restorative materials include amalgam, a variety of composite resins, and glass ionomers.

The continuous improvement in esthetic (tooth-colored) restorations has created growing demand by patients for restorative materials that match natural tooth shades. Because general dental practices spend a significant amount of time in the restoration of teeth, the dental assistant who is adept in the management, mixing, manipulation, and placement of chairside restorative materials is truly an asset to the dentist.

AMALGAM

Amalgam, like the other restorations described in this chapter, is a permanent restoration. Immediately following cavity preparation and placement of necessary liners and/or insulating bases, the dentist may place an amalgam restoration.

Use

Amalgam has been used as a permanent posterior restorative for many years because of its efficacy, relatively low cost, and durability. Amalgam is placed in posterior (back) teeth only because of its strength and ability to withstand chewing forces and because of its noticeable color (which would not present an esthetic appearance in anterior teeth).

Types of Alloy and Composition

Dental amalgam differs in types of alloy composition used. Metals comprising dental amalgam include (in descending order of content) silver, tin, copper, and sometimes zinc (see Table 4-1).

The ADA sets specific regulations regarding the composition of dental amalgam.

The alloy is mixed with mercury in a **triturator** (Figure 4-1A) to form the amalgam, which the dentist places into the cavity preparation. After placement it is condensed, carved, burnished, and polished. Figure 4-1B is an updated version of this machine.

Amalgam is supplied by manufacturers in lathe-cut and spherically shaped particles. The specific cut affects the properties and features.

Low-copper alloys are supplied with comminuted and spherical particles. High-copper alloys are supplied as comminuted, spherical, or combination particles.

Spherical alloys provide smoother surfaces that require a lower mercury content when amalgamated. Spherical alloys are easier to condense and provide improved carving and polishing properties. Combination alloys adapt more readily to the cavity preparation and produce better contacts with adjacent dentition.

Dental alloy is supplied in predispensed, disposable capsules. These capsules contain premeasured amounts of alloy, mercury, and a pestle separated by a plastic bubble barrier to prevent contact of the alloy and mercury prior to trituration. The pestle is a small plastic or metal pellet that helps mix the alloy and mercury at the appropriate time.

Components		Characteristics and Features:
Silver:	(40–70%) High-copper amalgam (68–72%) Low-copper mix	• Forms the metallic compound with mercury that determines dimensional changes that occur during set • Increases overall strength of the restoration • Increases expansion of the restoration • Requires slightly longer amalgamation • Sets quickly • Tarnishes easily • Decreases setting time
Tin:	(22–30%) High-copper amalgam (26–37%) Low-copper mix	• Helps in the amalgamation (chemical combination) of the alloy with mercury because of its high affinity for mercury • Reduces expansion during setting • Reduces strength • Sets more slowly • More susceptible to corrosion • Tends to weaken the restoration
Copper:	(12–30%) High-copper amalgam (4–5%) Low-copper mix	• Increases hardness and strength • Increases expansion of the amalgam during setting • Reduces flow of completed restoration • Resists corrosion (high copper) • Helps reduce marginal failure (high copper)
Zinc:	(0–1%) Both high- and low-copper amalgam	• Minimizes oxidation of metals during manufacture • Scavenges and reacts with oxygen to prevent it from combining with the other alloys • May cause excessive expansion if contacted by water (or saliva) during placement and manipulation

Table 4-1 Dental Alloy Composition: Components, Characteristics, and Features

Some capsules contain an activator that breaks the membrane or the capsules are twisted or compressed prior to trituration. Most disposable capsules are plastic and are supplied with a screw-type or friction-fit cap. Predispensed, disposable amalgam capsules are color coded to indicate single, double, or triple mixes (Figure 4–2).

The size of the mix corresponds to the size of the cavity preparation to receive the amalgam restoration; however, if the dentist is performing quadrant dentistry, multiple posterior teeth in the same quadrant or same side of the mouth may be prepared at the same appointment and multiple restorations placed at that time.

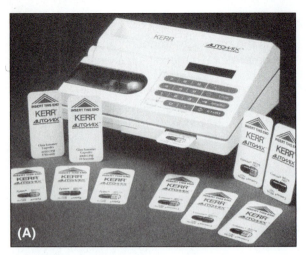

Figure 4-1A Triturator/amalgamator with individually predispensed amalgam capsules.

(Courtesy of Kerr Corporation.)

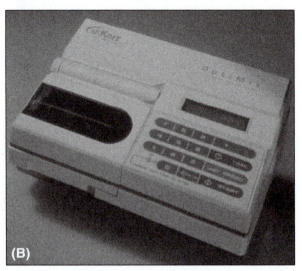

Figure 4-1B Optimix amalgamator.

(Courtesy of Kerr Corporation.)

Properties

Amalgam is used in posterior teeth due to its superior ability to withstand chewing forces. Skill in the manipulation of amalgam determines the outcome of the overall strength and long-term integrity of the restoration.

Amalgam is subject to dimensional changes, the most notable being expansion and contraction. The degree of expansion and

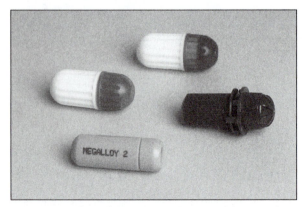

Figure 4-2 Predispensed, disposable amalgam capsules are color coded to indicate between single, double, and triple mixes.

contraction is controlled by the composition of the alloy and the dentist's manipulation techniques.

Amalgam restorations may also corrode, tarnish, or creep in the warm, moist, stressed environment of the oral cavity. Care and technique in finishing, carving, and polishing of amalgam restorations reduce corrosion and tarnish. Amalgam creep is a dimensional change that occurs in the material when it undergoes a constant load.

Mixing/Manipulation

The amalgam is mixed or triturated mechanically in a triturator, sometimes called an amalgamator. Amalgamation is the specific chemical reaction between the alloy and the mercury that forms the silver amalgam. A cradle holds the capsule. There are also a cradle cover, a timer, and a variable-speed control. The amalgamator must be set for the type of alloy used; trituration time is longer when larger amounts of restorative material are used. Most often, trituration is from 8 to 18 seconds (8 seconds for a one-spill capsule, 10–12 seconds for a two-spill, and 15–18 seconds for a three-spill capsule). The dental assistant should always follow the respective manufacturer's instructions when triturating amalgam.

The final quality of the amalgam restoration is dependent upon mixing time, speed, and force. An undertriturated mix may be crumbly and dull in appearance and the occlusal chewing strength will be compromised; an overtriturated mix may appear soupy before setting and may be difficult to remove from the capsule.

Amalgam Bonding

Amalgam bonding agents are used by some dentists to bond the amalgam material to the prepared tooth surface(s) (Figure 4–3). Benefits of amalgam bonding include

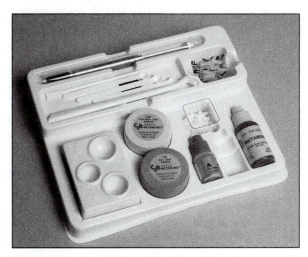

Figure 4-3 Amalgam bonding kit.

increased retention of the restoration and decreased marginal leakage.

Amalgam bonding agent is a low–viscosity resin, similar to those discussed in other chapters. Amalgam bonding takes place just prior to placing the amalgam restoration.

PRACTICE MAKES PERFECT PROCEDURE ▪ 4-1

Triturating Dental Amalgam

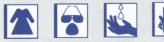

ARMAMENTARIUM
- Basic set-up
- High-speed amalgamator
- Predispensed, disposable amalgam capsule
- Amalgam well, dappen dish, or squeeze cloth
- Amalgam carrier
- Amalgam condenser(s)
- Covered scrap container for storing excess amalgam

PROCEDURE
1. Assemble required armamentarium for the procedure.
2. Prepare the predispensed amalgam capsule by twisting the cap, squeezing the capsule, or using the activator supplied by the manufacturer.
3. Insert the activated amalgam capsule into the cradle of the triturator, placing one end first, then sliding the other end down into place (Figure 4-4), using one hand.

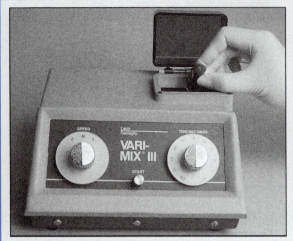

Figure 4-4 The dental assistant places the amalgam capsule into the cradle of the triturator.

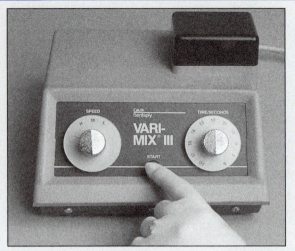

Figure 4-5 The dental assistant activates the amalgamator timer to triturate the mix.

4. Close the amalgamator cover. (The cover is a safety measure to help prevent mercury vapors from evaporating into the air and to prevent an errant capsule from flying out of the cradle accidentally during trituration.)

5. Activate the amalgamator (Figure 4-5) for the specified amount of time. (The amalgamator will automatically stop at the end of the timed cycle.)

6. Lift the cover and carefully remove the capsule, one end at a time.

7. Carefully open the capsule, taking care to avoid contacting the amalgam mix with the gloved hand, as this could contaminate the mix. Empty the contents of the capsule by gently tapping the material into an amalgam well or a dappen dish used especially for amalgam or onto a squeeze cloth. Use cotton pliers, if necessary, to remove the mix from the capsule.

8. Use the working edges of the capsule to scoop the pestle (if one is present inside the capsule) back into the capsule for disposal at the conclusion of the appointment. Screw or snap the used capsule closed and set it aside.

9. Place the index finger of the dominant hand underneath the flexible lever of the working end of the amalgam carrier and use a repetitive stroking or scraping motion to load either one or both ends of the

amalgam carrier (Figure 4-6). Most dentists have a preference as to whether the smaller or larger end is filled and used first. Pack or load the cylinder of the amalgam carrier tightly to avoid repetitive motions of filling and refilling the carrier. Wipe excess amalgam from the end or outside of the cylinder of the carrier onto the sides of the amalgam well or dappen dish or onto the squeeze cloth.

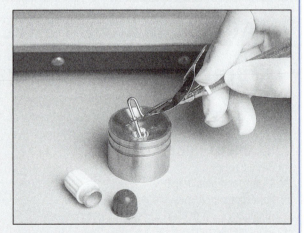

Figure 4-6 The dental assistant loads the amalgam carrier. Notice the positioning of the index finger.

10. Pass the filled amalgam carrier to the dentist and prepare to exchange it for the amalgam condenser. Repeat the instrument exchange and reloading of the amalgam carrier for as many times as directed by the dentist.

11. At the conclusion of amalgam placement into the cavity preparation, express excess amalgam from the cylinder of the amalgam carrier into a covered scrap amalgam container (Figure 4-7).

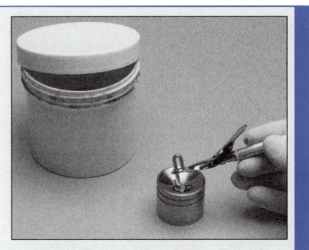

Figure 4-7 The dental assistant discards excess amalgam into a covered scrap container at the end of the procedure.

Special Considerations

- Express any remaining amalgam from the amalgam carrier immediately after use to prevent clogging.
- Store scrap and excess amalgam in a covered container.
- Always wear PPE when working at chairside.
- Maintain and work in a clean, dry, aseptic field.
- Clean and disinfect the work area at the conclusion of the procedure, after dismissing the patient.
- Always follow OSHA regulations and CDC recommendations to help prevent the spread of bloodborne diseases and to protect dental personnel.

■ MERCURY

Mercury, used in the **trituration** (mixing) of alloy to form amalgam restorations, has long been known to be a health hazard to those who ingest, contact, or inhale its vapors for prolonged periods. Excessive exposure to mercury has been associated with mental impairment, skin rashes, and spontaneous miscarriage.

Mercury is a metal in liquid form used to wet dry alloy particles. Upon condensing, the mercury-rich layer rises to the surface from the cavity preparation and is then carved off or aspirated from the restoration by the chairside assistant. Approximately only 3 percent of the mercury is left in an amalgam restoration.

However, in the amounts used in amalgam restorations, mercury is extremely minimal and as such should not pose an occupational health risk to members of the dental team or patients if handled following proper guidelines (Box 4-1).

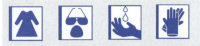

The assistant who selects, handles, mixes, manipulates, transfers, and disposes of silver amalgam material should follow these guidelines for safe mercury management:

1. Work in well-ventilated operatories.
2. Avoid direct skin contact with mercury—always wear gloves during patient care.
3. Never inhale mercury vapors. The dental assistant who must handle mercury should do so over a tray, which will help contain an accidental spill.
4. Use predispensed capsules in an amalgamator with a cover that prevents mercury vapor from escaping during trituration. (Always close the cover before and during trituration.) Close capsule as soon as it is emptied.
5. Use high-volume evacuation when finishing or removing amalgam restorations. Evacuation systems should have traps or filters. Check and clean or replace disposable traps and filters periodically.
6. Store mercury in unbreakable, tightly sealed containers away from heat sources. (A tightly fitted cover keeps potentially harmful mercury vapors from escaping into the air.) Research demonstrates that gelatine or glycerine also prevent mercury vapors from escaping from a sealed jar of scrap amalgam.
7. Salvage scrap amalgam by storing it under photographic or dental x-ray fixer solution or submerging it in a solution of bleach and water in a tightly closed, unbreakable container. (Water alone is inadequate for this purpose.)
8. Clean up spilled mercury using appropriate procedures and equipment, such as a mercury spill kit (Figure 4-8); do not use bare hands or a household vacuum cleaner.
9. Where feasible, recycle scrap amalgam and waste amalgam. Otherwise, dispose of amalgam scrap and waste amalgam in accordance with applicable local laws.
10. Place contaminated disposable mercury-containing materials in double-sealed, polyethylene bags for proper disposal.
11. Apply a biohazard sticker or label to the waste bag.

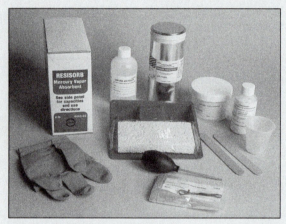

Figure 4-8 Mercury spill kit.

Box 4-1 Guidelines for Handling Mercury Safely

Mercury Hygiene

All members of the dental team should be trained in the proper handling and potential hazards of mercury vapor as well as the necessity of observing sound mercury hygiene practices.

The ADA states that mercury-containing amalgam is a safe, economical, and effective restorative material and that there is no scientific evidence that exposure to mercury from amalgam restorations poses a serious health risk in humans, except for the exceedingly small number of allergic reactions.

The FDA concludes there is no reason to routinely remove amalgam fillings for replacement with composite or gold restorations.

Burnishing of the amalgam restoration after the final carving removes most of the excess mercury from the patient's oral cavity. Scrap amalgam may be safely stored using a scrap mercury container with the contents kept covered to prevent the release of mercury vapors and the mercury submerged completely in photoprocessing or x-ray fixer solution or a solution of bleach and water.

As with all hazardous substances, mercury should be handled carefully, which includes proper labeling, keeping a **Material Safety Data Sheet (MSDS)** on file, and proper disposal.

How to Clean Up a Mercury Spill

In the event that a mercury spill occurs, the dental assistant should follow the recommended guidelines for cleaning up the spill (Box 4-2).

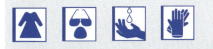

In the event of a mercury spill, the dental assistant should follow these guidelines:

1. If a spill occurs on a carpeted floor, do not use a vacuum cleaner or bare hands to collect it.
2. Pick up all visible droplets of spilled mercury with narrow-bore tubing connected by a wash bottle trap to a low-volume aspirator on the dental unit. The trap bottle connections will keep the mercury in the bottle and prevent it from being sucked back into the dental unit.
3. Use adhesive tape to clean up small spills.
4. If the spilled mercury droplets are not easily within reach, dust them with sulfur powder, which will form a film coating on the top of the mercury droplets.
5. Keep a commercial mercury spill kit on hand. Follow the manufacturer's directions and document the circumstances of the accidental spill with the date and clean-up measures used.

Box 4-2 Recommended Guidelines for Cleaning a Mercury Spill

■ COMPOSITE

Composite restorative material is an alternative to amalgam, due largely to its property of matching natural tooth shades. It is less dense than amalgam, however. A composite restoration is placed into a prepared tooth and then self-cured, light cured, or dual cured. The light-cured single-paste system contains a photoinitiator and an amine activator supplied in disposable light-proof syringes (Figure 4-9).

Composite restorative material is supplied in syringes or in single-application cartridges (compules) in a variety of tooth-matching shades.

Once the composite material is placed in the prepared tooth, polymerization is achieved by shining a small beam of visible blue light onto the restoration for approximately 20–30 seconds.

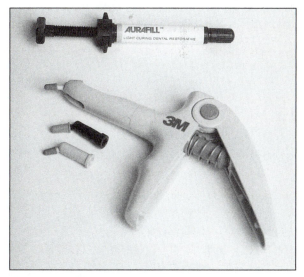

Figure 4-9 Composite syringes and cartridges.

All composite restoratives contain the following components:
- An organic polymer matrix, such as BIS-GMA or urethane dimethacrylate
- Inorganic filler particles, such as lithium aluminum silicate, quartz, or silica
- Organic silane coupling agents treated with a coupling agent to create a bond between the first two components

Box 4-3 Contents of Composites

Use

Composite restorations, first used for anterior restorations only because of their esthetic appearance, are now used for both anterior and posterior restorations. Another advantage is that no mercury is required, as with amalgam, for patients who have a desire to avoid contact with mercury.

Composition

Composite filling materials vary in composition depending upon their content and intended use (see Box 4-3). Their classification depends upon the type, amount, and size of the filler particles. The particles may be fine, microfill, or a combination of the fine and microfill, called hybrids (see Table 4-2). These filler particles, which add strength to the finished restoration, may comprise up to 84 percent of the composite material volume. Polishability is directly related to particle size.

Properties

Properties of composite restorations vary depending upon the content and manufacturer and the size of the filler particles (see Box 4-4).

Mixing/Manipulation

The finished cavity preparation is acid etched for 30–60 seconds prior to placing the composite restoration. Then the dental assistant uses the air/water syringe to completely rinse and dry the prepared tooth surface. The tooth will have a chalky or frosted appearance, which indicates that etching has been effective.

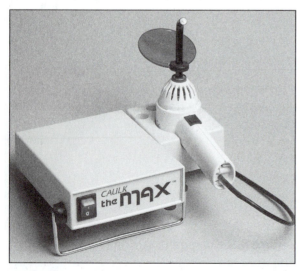

Figure 4-10 Visible blue-light curing system.

Fine composites (called macrofill)

- Contain filler particles from 1 to 3 μm
- Are often utilized for Class IV restorations due to their strength to resist fractures
- Are esthetically pleasing for anterior teeth
- Do not take as high a polish as microfills and hybrids

Microfill composites

- Contain fillers from 0.01 to 0.1 μm
- Are used in Class III and Class V restorations
- Are used for direct veneers and diastema closures
- May be used for Class IV and the occlusal portion of Class I and Class II restoration
- Are esthetic and resist wear from abrasion
- Take a high polish

Hybrid composites

- Contain glass and silica filler particles
- Are stronger and less likely to fracture than microfill composites
- Combine the strength and esthetics of macrofill and microfill composites
- Provide a restoration that is strong and polishable

Table 4-2 Types of Composites and Features

Etching is performed to increase bonding strength between the composite and the tooth surface, which increases retention and decreases marginal leakage. Adhesion of the composite can be further improved by using a bonding agent.

General properties of composite restorations may include the following:
- Fracture resistance
- Improved resistance to occlusal wear
- Esthetics that match natural tooth color and opacity
- Addition of a radiopaquing material to some composites that makes the restoration (and the margin) more visible on radiographs
- Efficient bonding capacity to dentin and enamel
- May require placement/application in layers to reduce polymerization-related shrinkage
- Smooth finish
- Improved strength to withstand occlusal wear
- Expansion and contraction rates similar to natural tooth structure

Box 4-4 General Properties of Composites

Using the two-paste, self-curing system, the dental assistant dispenses and mixes equal amounts of catalyst paste and base onto a paper mixing pad, close to but not touching each other. Upon the direction of the dentist, the assistant incorporates one into the other, completing spatulation within 30 seconds.

The dentist usually applies the composite material in layers to help minimize shrinkage of the composite. Immediately after each layer is placed in the prepared tooth, the material is light cured to the desired hardness (unless a self-curing system is used).

■ GLASS IONOMER RESTORATIONS

Type II glass ionomer materials (also known as compomers) may also be used where the dentist and patient prefer an esthetic restoration that does not require high compression

Mixing Composite Material: Two-Paste, Self-Curing

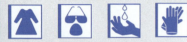

ARMAMENTARIUM

- Basic set-up
- Composite base paste
- Catalyst paste
- Paper mixing pad (supplied by the manufacturer)
- Disposable plastic spatula (supplied by the manufacturer)
- Plastic placement instrument
- A curing light for single-paste systems
- 2 × 2 gauze sponges

PROCEDURE

1. Assemble required armamentarium for the procedure.
2. Using opposite ends of the (marked) plastic mixing spatula, dispense equal (small) amounts of base and catalyst paste onto the mixing pad. Note: The dental assistant should take great care to avoid touching one material to the other because this will initiate polymerization (hardening) and will risk contaminating the entire contents of the jar.
3. Using the same spatula, mix the base paste and catalyst together, usually within 30 seconds. The mix will exhibit a dough consistency. Note that the composite material begins to polymerize almost immediately. Do not overmix or manipulate.
4. Gather the mixed composite material into a mass on the mixing pad and deliver it near the patient's chin, out of the patient's line of vision, and hold the mixing pad for the dentist to use.
5. Pass a plastic instrument to the dentist for placing the mixed composite into the cavity preparation.
6. After the dentist has placed the composite, be prepared to receive the plastic placement instrument. Use a 2 × 2 gauze to immediately wipe any excess composite left on the instrument. (This saves clean-up time later.)
7. At the completion of the procedure discard the top sheet of the mixing pad and the disposable mixing spatula.

Special Considerations

- Take great care to prevent contaminating the mix; to avoid this, use opposite ends of the mixing spatula when dispensing the composite material.
- When working with composites, always use plastic mixing spatulas (sticks) and placement instruments because the material will adhere to metal instruments and become very difficult to remove.
- Always wear PPE when working at chairside.
- Maintain and work in a clean, dry, aseptic field.
- Clean and disinfect the work area at the conclusion of the procedure, after dismissing the patient.
- Always follow OSHA regulations and CDC recommendations to help prevent the spread of bloodborne diseases and to protect dental personnel.

Composite Restoration: Syringe-Type Material

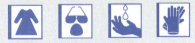

ARMAMENTARIUM

- Basic set-up
- Composite syringe and compules
- Plastic placement instrument
- 2 × 2 gauze sponges

PROCEDURE

1. Assemble required armamentarium for the procedure.
2. Determine the shade for composite. Record the shade on the patient's chart for future reference.
3. When the cavity preparation is complete, rinse and dry the preparation.
4. Transfer a brush or applicator tip containing the acid-etching materials to the dentist. The dentist will then apply the acid etch to the cavity preparation. Carefully read the manufacturer's directions and inform the dentist of the length of time the material must remain on the tooth. Then rinse the tooth thoroughly after the recommended time.
5. Read the manufacturer's instruction's carefully and ensure that the adhesive or bonding material is placed according to those instructions. Some bonding materials require that the assistant use the curing light to set the bonding material. With some bonding resins, a primer or conditioner is placed before the bonding material.
6. Ensure that composites are applied with a single-application syringe and compule tip or a syringe which has composite material for many applications. The material may be placed directly into the cavity preparation. Some dentists may use a composite placement instrument to assist in the placement of the composite material. The material is placed in incremental layers and light cured after each layer is placed. This ensures that each layer is cured.
7. Check the occlusion with articulating paper. The dentist will remove any high areas indicated by the articulating paper.
8. Rinse the patient's mouth to ensure that pieces of the composite material do not remain.

Special Considerations

- Always wipe off the metal spatula and plastic instrument with a 2 × 2 gauze as soon as the cement has been used to make clean-up easier.
- Always wear PPE when working at chairside.
- Maintain and work in a clean, dry, aseptic field.
- Clean and disinfect the work area at the conclusion of the procedure, after dismissing the patient.
- Always follow OSHA regulations and CDC recommendations to help prevent the spread of bloodborne diseases and to protect dental personnel.

strength and where amalgam may be unsightly (providing only fair esthetics). Glass ionomer as a cement and dentin replacement (base) are addressed in Chapter 3. Students are advised to review that portion of the chapter before proceeding.

Type II glass ionomer restorative is supplied as powder and liquid, as paste systems, in syringes, and in capsule forms. Glass ionomers are also supplied in either self-curing or light-curing systems.

Use

Because Type II glass ionomers are not as strong as most composites, they are most often used for non-stress-bearing restorations, such as Class V restorations (for treating root caries) on the gingival one-third area and for Class III (anterior interproximal restorations). Type II ionomers are indicated for primary tooth restoration because they also contain time-released fluoride.

Composition

Combining composite resins with glass ionomers has markedly improved the qualities of glass ionomer restoration. These materials are supplied with tooth-matching shades and light cured. Glass ionomer powder is a silicate glass powder containing calcium, aluminum,

---

PRACTICE MAKES PERFECT PROCEDURE ▪ 4-4

Glass Ionomer Restorative Material

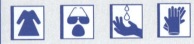

ARMAMENTARIUM
- Basic set-up
- Glass ionomer cement powder and scoop (dispenser)
- Glass ionomer liquid
- Paper mixing pad (or cooled glass slab)
- Cement spatula
- 2 × 2 gauze sponges (moistened with a 10% sodium hydroxide solution)
- Minute timer
- Plastic instrument

PROCEDURE
1. For mixing procedure, refer to Practice Makes Perfect Procedure 3-6: Mixing Glass Ionomer Cement in Chapter 3.
2. Apply calcium hydroxide to the deepest areas of the cavity preparation.
3. Apply tooth conditioner to the dentin for 10 seconds to remove the smear layer.
4. Rinse the tooth with a steady flow of water for 30 seconds.
5. Dry the tooth using a gentle stream of air, taking care not to dehydrate the tooth tissues.
6. Apply base to cover dentin, including the dentino-enamel junction. Allow the base to set for 2 minutes.
7. Acid etch the enamel using etching gel or liquid for 30 seconds.
8. Rinse the tooth with a steady stream of water for 60 seconds.
9. Dry the tooth again with a gentle stream of air, taking care not to dehydrate it.
10. Place the glass ionomer restorative material.
11. Place a protective sealant or enamel bonding agent.

---

and fluoride (calcium fluoroaluminosilicate glass). The liquid is an aqueous solution of polyacrylic acid. Glass ionomer cement is available as a powder and liquid system and in capsules. The capsules require a high-speed amalgamator to mix the cement.

Properties

Glass ionomer restorations pass through two setting stages; the filling material must be protected against moisture contamination and dehydration. Glass ionomers are nonirritating. Complete setting time takes up to 24 hours.

Mixing/Manipulation

Placement and manipulation of glass ionomer restorations are similar to those of composite materials with only a few exceptions. The dentist prepares the tooth more conservatively without mechanical retention or bevels. Sometimes, the dentist will apply retraction cord subgingivally to control gingival hemorrhage (which might contaminate the tooth-colored restoration with moisture from saliva and blood).

Glass ionomer restoratives can be mixed on either a paper mixing pad or a cool glass slab. A paper mixing pad is desirable because of ease and speed of clean-up; however, a cooled glass slab may be used to retard working and/or setting time.

The powder is fluffed prior to dispensing, then measured out using the scoop (dispenser) supplied by the manufacturer. Then the liquid is dispensed prior to spatulation. Mixing time is 30–60 seconds. Setting time is approximately 5 minutes.

The prepared tooth is cleansed using a chlorhexidine soap solution. Finishing and polishing of glass ionomers may require special lubricants. The dentist may apply a layer of light-cured enamel bonding agent or pit and fissure sealant over the finished glass ionomer restoration.

■ CRITICAL THINKING QUESTIONS

1. Why should the chairside dental assistant express any remaining amalgam from the amalgam carrier cylinder immediately after the dentist is finished using it?
2. Why is scrap amalgam stored in a covered container?
3. Why should plastic spatulas and placement instruments (only) be used when mixing and placing composite restorative materials?
4. What limitations do glass ionomer restoratives have?

PRACTICE MAKES PERFECT
STUDENT ASSESSMENT 4-1

Triturating Dental Amalgam

Student's Name: _____

Date: _____ Instructor: _____

Note: The blank space is provided for the instructor to check off the student's progress. The student may practice the procedure as many times as necessary before being evaluated. Some portions of the exercise may be performed on a typodont, stone tooth model, or extracted tooth or simulated in a clinical operatory. The student has successfully completed the following:

_____ Worn necessary PPE

_____ Assembled necessary armamentarium

_____ Maintained a clear, dry, aseptic working field

_____ Prepared the predispensed amalgam capsule by twisting the cap, squeezing the capsule, or using the activator supplied by the manufacturer

_____ Inserted the activated amalgam capsule into the cradle of the triturator, placing one end first, then sliding the other end down into place, using one hand

_____ Closed the amalgamator cover

_____ Activated the amalgamator for the specified amount of time

_____ Lifted the cover and carefully removed the capsule, one end at a time

_____ Carefully opened the capsule, taking care to avoid contacting the amalgam mix with the gloved hand

_____ Emptied the contents of the capsule by gently tapping the material into an amalgam well or dappen dish or onto a squeeze cloth and use cotton pliers, if necessary, to remove the mix from the capsule

_____ Used the working edges of the capsule to scoop the pestle (if one is present inside the capsule) back into the capsule for disposal at the conclusion of the appointment and screwed or snapped the used capsule closed and set it aside

_____ Placed the index finger of the dominant hand underneath the flexible lever of the working end of the amalgam carrier and used a repetitive stroking or scraping motion to load both ends of the amalgam carrier

_____ Packed the cylinder of the amalgam carrier tightly to avoid repetitive motions of filling and refilling the carrier

_____ Wiped excess amalgam from the end or outside of the cylinder of the carrier onto the sides of the amalgam well or dappen dish or onto the squeeze cloth

_____ Passed the filled amalgam carrier to the dentist and prepared to exchange it for the amalgam condenser

_____ Repeated the instrument exchange and reloaded the amalgam carrier for as many times as directly by the dentist

_____ At the conclusion of amalgam placement into the cavity preparation, expressed excess amalgam from the cylinder of the amalgam carrier into a covered scrap amalgam container and replaced the cover

_____ Cleaned and disinfected the work area at the conclusion of the procedure, after dismissing the patient

_____ Followed OSHA regulations and CDC recommendations to help prevent the spread of bloodborne diseases and to protect dental personnel

Comments

_____

_____

_____

_____

_____

Mixing Composite Material: Two-Paste, Self-Curing

Student's Name _____

Date: _____   Instructor: _____

Note: The blank space is provided for the instructor to check off the student's progress. The student may practice the procedure as many times as necessary before being evaluated. Some portions of the exercise may be performed on a typodont, stone tooth model, or extracted tooth or simulated in a clinical operatory. The student has successfully completed the following:

_____ Worn necessary PPE

_____ Assembled necessary armamentarium

_____ Maintained a clear, dry, aseptic working field

_____ Used opposite ends of the (marked) plastic mixing spatula and dispensed equal (small) amounts of base and catalyst paste onto the mixing to avoid contamination

_____ Mixed the base paste and catalyst together within 30 seconds

_____ Gathered the mixed composite material into a mass on the mixing pad and delivered it near to the patient's chin, out of the patient's line of vision, and held it there for the dentist to use

_____ Passed the dentist a plastic instrument for placing the mixed composite into the cavity preparation

_____ Received the plastic placement instrument

_____ Used a 2 × 2 gauze to immediately wipe any excess composite left on the instrument

_____ At the completion of the procedure, discarded the top sheet of the mixing pad and the disposable mixing spatula

_____ Cleaned and disinfected the work area at the conclusion of the procedure, after dismissing the patient

_____ Followed OSHA regulations and CDC recommendations to help prevent the spread of bloodborne diseases and to protect dental personnel

Comments

_____

_____

_____

_____

_____

PRACTICE MAKES PERFECT
STUDENT ASSESSMENT 4-3

Composite Restoration: Syringe-Type Material

Student's Name: _____

Date: _____   Instructor: _____

Note: The blank space is provided for the instructor to check off the student's progress. The student may practice the procedure as many times as necessary before being evaluated. Some portions of the exercise may be performed on a typodont, stone tooth model, or extracted tooth or simulated in a clinical operatory. The student has successfully completed the following:

_____ Worn necessary PPE

_____ Assembled necessary armamentarium

_____ Maintained a clear, dry, aseptic working field

_____ Determined the shade for the composite

_____ Recorded the shade on the patient's chart for future reference

_____ When the cavity preparation is complete, rinsed and dried the preparation

_____ Transferred a brush or applicator tip containing the acid-etching materials to the dentist

_____ Read the manufacturer's directions and informed the dentist of the length of time the material must remain on the tooth

_____ Rinsed the tooth thoroughly after the recommended time

_____ Ensured that the adhesive or bonding material was placed according to the manufacturer's instructions

_____ Passed composites to the dentist

_____ Passed a composite placement instrument to the dentist to assist in the placement of the composite material, if necessary

_____ Light cured the material after each layer was placed to ensure that each layer was cured

_____ Passed the dentist the articulating paper to check the occlusion

_____ Wiped off any remaining marks left by the articulating paper with a 2 × 2 gauze

_____ Rinsed the patient's mouth to ensure that pieces of the composite material did not remain

_____ Cleaned and disinfected the work area at the conclusion of the procedure, after dismissing the patient

_____ Followed OSHA regulations and CDC recommendations to help prevent the spread of bloodborne diseases and to protect dental personnal

Comments

_____

_____

_____

_____

_____

Glass Ionomer Restorative Material

Student's Name: _____

Date: _____   Instructor: _____

Note: The blank space is provided for the instructor to check off the student's progress. The student may practice the procedure as many times as necessary before being evaluated. Some portions of the exercise may be performed on a typodont, stone tooth model, or extracted tooth or simulated in a clinical operatory. The student has successfully completed the following:

_____ Worn necessary PPE

_____ Assembled necessary armamentarium

_____ Maintained a clear, dry, aseptic working field

_____ Applied calcium hydroxide to the deepest areas of the cavity preparation

_____ Applied tooth conditioner to the dentin for 10 seconds to remove the smear layer

_____ Rinsed the tooth with a steady flow of water for 30 seconds

_____ Dried the tooth using a gentle stream of air, taking care not to dehydrate the tooth tissues

_____ Applied base to cover dentin, including the dentinoenamel junction and allowed the base to set for 2 minutes

_____ Acid etched the enamel using etching gel or liquid for 30 seconds

_____ Rinsed the tooth with a steady stream of water for 60 seconds

_____ Dried the tooth again with a gentle stream of air, taking care not to dehydrate it

_____ Placed the glass ionomer restorative material

_____ Placed a protective sealant or enamel bonding agent

_____ Cleaned and disinfected the work area at the conclusion of the procedure, after dismissing the patient

_____ Followed OSHA regulations and CDC recommendations to help prevent the spread of bloodborne diseases and to protect dental personnel

Comments

_____

_____

_____

_____

_____

CHAPTER 4: POSTTEST

Instructions: For each of the following, select the answer that most accurately completes the question or statement.

1. All of the following statements are true of amalgam *except*
    A. Amalgam has been used as a permanent posterior restorative for many years because of its efficacy and durability.
    B. Amalgam has been used as a permanent posterior restorative for many years because of its relatively low cost.
    C. Amalgam is used in both anterior and posterior teeth.
    D. Amalgam is placed in posterior (back) teeth only because of its strength and ability to withstand chewing forces.

2. Amalgam restorations may contain all of the following *except*
    A. silver
    B. tin
    C. copper
    D. composite
    E. zinc

3. _____, a significant component of dental alloy, forms the metallic compound with mercury that determines dimensional changes that occur during set.
    A. Zinc
    B. Silver
    C. Tin
    D. Copper

4. _____ increases hardness, strength, and expansion of amalgam during setting.
    A. Zinc
    B. Silver
    C. Tin
    D. Copper

5. _____ scavenges and reacts with oxygen to prevent it from combining with the other alloys.
    A. Zinc
    B. Silver
    C. Tin
    D. Copper

6. A premeasured, predispensed amalgam capsule may contain all of the following *except*
    A. mercury
    B. alloy
    C. glass ionomer
    D. pestle
    E. membrane

7. Dental amalgam may be subject to all of the following changes *except*
   A. expansion and contraction
   B. corrosion
   C. tarnish
   D. creep
   E. pulp insulation

8. The cover on an amalgamator is a safety measure designed to
   A. help prevent mercury vapors from evaporating into the air
   B. prevent an errant capsule from flying out of the cradle accidentally during trituration
   C. help clean up an amalgam spill
   D. A and B only
   E. B and C only

9. The amount of mercury used in amalgam restorations is extremely minimal and as such should not pose an occupational health risk to members of the dental team or to patients if handled following proper guidelines.
   A. True
   B. False

10. In the event of a mercury spill, the dental assistant should clean it up using
    A. his or her bare hands
    B. a household vacuum cleaner
    C. a mercury spill kit
    D. x-ray fixer solution

11. The FDA recommends the routine removal of amalgam fillings for replacement with composite or gold restorations.
    A. True
    B. False

12. All of the following are true regarding composite restorative material *except*
    A. It is an alternative to amalgam.
    B. It has the property of matching natural tooth shades.
    C. It is denser than amalgam.
    D. It may be supplied in self-cured, light-cured, or dual-cured systems.

13. Once the composite material is placed in the prepared tooth, polymerization is achieved by shining a small beam of visible blue light onto the restoration for approximately _____ seconds.
    A. 10–15
    B. 15–20
    C. 20–30
    D. 30–60

14. Mixing time for two-paste, self-curing composite should take place within _____ seconds.
    A. 10
    B. 20
    C. 30
    D. 60

15. To avoid permanent eye damage, the dentist and chairside dental assistant should always wear light-filtering protective eye shields or use a light-screening safety tip when using visible blue light.
    A. True
    B. False

16. Composite restorations may be indicated for all of the following *except*
    A. use in anterior teeth due to their esthetic appearance
    B. use in posterior teeth in some instances
    C. for patients who desire to avoid contact with mercury
    D. for root canal filling material

17. Organic silane coupling agents create a bond between polymer matrix, such as BIS-GMA, and inorganic filler particles to form composite restorative material.
    A. True
    B. False

18. _____ are used in Class III, Class IV, and Class V restorations and take a high polish.
    A. Fine composites
    B. Microfill composites
    C. Hybrid composites
    D. Amalgam restorations

19. All of the following are general properties of composites *except*
    A. Composites are fracture resistant.
    B. Composites provide esthetic matching to natural tooth color and opacity.
    C. Some composites contain a radiopaquing material, which makes them more visible on radiographs.
    D. Composites bond efficiently to dentin and enamel.
    E. Due to their exothermic reaction during spatulation, composites must be mixed on a glass slab.

20. After placing a glass ionomer restoration, the dentist may apply a layer of light-cured enamel bonding agent or pit and fissure sealant over the completed restoration.
    A. True
    B. False

SECTION · III

Impression Materials

Chapter 5 Dental Impression Materials

To be tolerant with my associates, for at times I too make mistakes.

To be friendly, realizing that friendship bestows and receives happiness.

To be respectful of the other person's viewpoint and condition.

Excerpt from the "Creed for Dental Assistants" by Juliette A. Southard.
Reprinted with the permission of the American Dental Assistants Association, Chicago, IL.

DENTAL IMPRESSION MATERIALS ▪ CHAPTER 5

LEARNING OBJECTIVES

Upon completion of this chapter the student should be able to:

1. Describe the general types of impression materials used in dentistry and their specific applications.

2. Describe the role and duties of the dental assistant in the use, instrumentation, manipulation, application, and clean-up procedures required when working with hydrocolloid impression (irreversible and reversible) materials.

3. Describe the role and duties of the dental assistant in the use, instrumentation, manipulation, application, and clean-up procedures required when working with polysulfide elastomeric impression materials.

4. Describe the role and duties of the dental assistant in the use, instrumentation, manipulation, application, and clean-up procedures required when working with condensation silicone and addition polysiloxane/polyvinyl elastomeric impression materials.

5. Describe the role and duties of the dental assistant in the use, instrumentation, manipulation, application, and clean-up procedures required when working with polyether impression materials.

6. Describe the role and duties of the dental assistant in disinfection of various dental impression materials.

7. Describe the role and duties of the dental assistant in procedures required when working with bite registration paste.

KEY TERMS

gel
hydrocolloid
polyether
polymerization

polysiloxane/polyvinyl
polysulfide/rubber base
retarder
sol

■ INTRODUCTION

The well-trained dental assistant is an asset to the dentist in assisting with chairside and laboratory-related procedures. Familiarity and skill in the mixing, manipulation, and follow-up laboratory procedures required when working with a wide variety of impression materials makes the dental assistant a valued member of the dental team.

As with restorative materials (Chapter 4: Restorative Dental Materials), dental impression materials are supplied by a wide variety of manufacturers, each with specific directions for storage, shelf life, manipulation, and use. Prior to working with any impression material, the dental assistant is advised to review the specific manufacturer's directions and related packing materials.

Instructions for mixing, manipulation, and use of various impression materials described in this chapter are a compilation of various methods. The dental assistant should note that each dental practitioner may have specific preferences for methods and procedures.

■ HYDROCOLLOID IMPRESSION MATERIAL (IRREVERSIBLE)

Impressions are used in dentistry to make an accurate reproduction of the teeth, dental arches, and related supporting hard and soft structures. Irreversible **hydrocolloid** impressions (often referred to as alginate) are one of the most commonly used types of impressions in the dental office.

An alginate impression is a primary, less accurate impression which is then poured in a gypsum (plaster or stone) cast or study model (see Chapter 6: Dental Gypsum Materials for further information). The alginate impression creates a "negative" impression of the area of the mouth the dentist directs to be duplicated, and then poured in stone, which sets and is then separated from the alginate impression to reveal the "positive" replication.

Alginate is referred to as irreversible because once the material is spatulated and used to make an oral impression, it cannot be returned to its original state. It is used only once and discarded.

Use

Alginate impressions are used routinely in dentistry to make upper and lower study models for fixed and removable prosthetics, orthodontic appliances, mouth guards, bleaching trays (stents), provisional restorations, and custom acrylic trays.

Composition

Alginate irreversible impression material is made from potassium alginate, which is an extract of seaweed (kelp). It also contains flavoring and may be white or have pastel coloring added to increase patient acceptance. Added to this is calcium sulfate, which, through a chemical reaction, forms a **gel**.

Trisodium phosphate is added as a **retarder** to control setting time and to allow for the material to be placed into the tray and into the patient's oral cavity. (A retarder slows the setting time.) Fillers, including diatomaceous earth and zinc oxide, are also added to alginate powder to make up the bulk of the material (50–75 percent).

Some manufacturers add a small amount of potassium titanium fluoride to the alginate powder to counteract the tendency of the material to soften the surface of gypsum products upon contact with the alginate.

Properties

Alginate powder is supplied in cans or predispensed packets (Figure 5-1); it dissolves quickly in water to form a viscous **sol**. There are a number of advantages and disadvantages of using alginate impression material (see Table 5-1).

Mixing/Manipulation

Gelation time is the time from which the alginate powder is mixed with water until it sets completely. This gelation time differs according to the type of alginate used. Type I is fast setting; Type II is regular setting.

Gelation time depends upon two factors: the working time and the setting time. Working time refers to the time required for the dental assistant to spatulate the material, load it into the impression tray, and insert it into the patient's upper or lower arch. Setting time is the time at which the mixed alginate

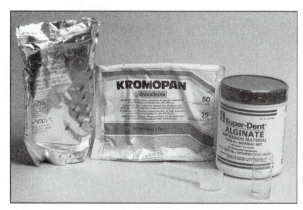

Figure 5-1 Foil bags and plastic canister of alginate irreversible impression material (powder) with measuring devices.

impression material begins to set through a chemical reaction until it is completely set and is ready to be removed from the oral cavity (see Table 5-2).

Setting time can be altered by increasing or decreasing or by adjusting the temperature of the water used to mix the alginate. The suggested temperature should be room temperature [70°F (21°C)]. As the water temperature increases, the working time decreases. If the

---

Advantages

- Ease of mixing and manipulation
- Minimal equipment and armamentarium required
- Economical to use
- Meets most accuracy requirements for primary casts
- Rapid set
- Affords patient comfort
- Usable for soft- and hard-tissue impressions
- Elastic properties that allow ease of withdrawal (removal) from undercuts found in the oral cavity

Disadvantages

- Loss of accuracy from atmospheric conditions (e.g., humidity)
- Thickened consistency that can cause minimal tissue distortion
- Less precise than secondary impression materials

Table 5-1 Alginate Irreversible Impression Material: Advantages and Disadvantages

Alginate Type	Working Time	Setting Time
Type I alginate (fast set)	60 seconds	1–2 minutes
Type II alginate (regular set)	2–4$\frac{1}{2}$ minutes	2–4$\frac{1}{2}$ minutes

Table 5-2 Working and Setting Times for Alginate Irreversible Impression Material

humidity and room temperature increase, the working time may also decrease, especially in warm, humid climates.

Alginate powder should be stored in its original, sealed container until ready for use. Storage temperatures in excess of 120°F may cause loss of strength and lowered resistance to deformity. If stored in highly moist conditions, the material may demonstrate inconsistent setting time. The powder should be stored in a cool, dry place, with the lid kept tightly in place when not in use. It should be kept no longer than one year.

The manufacturers of alginate impression material supply water- and powder-measuring devices, which should be used with the respective manufacturer's impression material. The dental assistant should always read and follow the manufacturer's directions; for example, the powder may need to be fluffed prior to opening or the powder may need to be packed into the measuring scoop when dispensing it.

The water-measuring device is a plastic cylinder with lines that indicate the amount of water to be used for each scoop of powder. Two scoops of powder and two increments of water are required for each mandibular full-arch impression. Three scoops of powder and three increments of water are required for each maxillary full-arch impression. This is because the maxillary arch impression includes the surface area of the hard palate.

Alginate impression material may be mixed in single-use disposable mixing bowls and with spatulas (or tongue depressors) or in reusable rubber mixing bowls and spatulas (Figure 5-2). The alginate is spatulated (stropped) along the side of the bowl over a wide space with wide, sweeping strokes to incorporate the powder into the water and to eliminate air bubbles.

The operator will indicate a preference for the type of tray required (Figure 5-3).

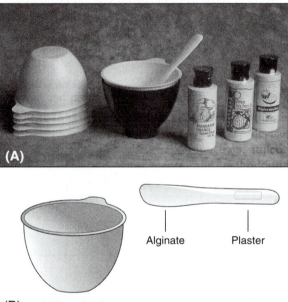

(A)

Alginate   Plaster

(B)   Alginate bowl

Figure 5-2 Examples of disposable and reusable bowls and spatulas the dental assistant uses to mix alginate. (A) Bowl-Away and Spat-Away are disposable bowls used to mix alginate and plaster. (B) Bowl-Away and Spat-Away indicate the water measuring lines in the mixing bowl. The opposite ends of the spatula are for use as indicated. *(Courtesy of Direct Crown LLC.)*

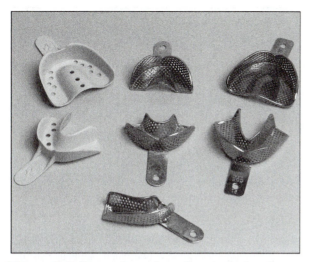

Figure 5-3 Examples of perforated plastic (disposable) and metal (autoclavable and reusable) alginate impression trays.

Alginate trays are made of either plastic or metal and contain holes, through which the alginate material will ooze and lock into the tray for complete removal after the setting time has been completed. (Otherwise, the impression material would remain attached to the oral tissues when the tray is removed.) Several trays should be tried in the patient's mouth prior to starting to mix the alginate. This helps the patient acclimate to the procedure and to be better prepared to know what to expect. The tray should extend 2–3 mm past the last molar and below both the lingual and facial surfaces of the teeth. In some instances, wax must be placed to extend the periphery of the tray.

Note that when both maxillary and mandibular impressions are required, the mandibular impression is taken first. This is to introduce the patient to the impression procedure as well as because patients are more likely to experience a gag reflex when the maxillary impression is taken. To help the patient with a gag reflex, the dental assistant may have the patient rinse with cold water prior to the impression or spray a topical anesthetic on the patient's hard and soft palate (for maxillary impressions).

In some states, the dental assistant is legally allowed to take alginate impressions under the supervision of the dentist because the procedure is considered reversible; in other states only the dentist may take and remove alginate (or any other type of impressions) from the oral cavity.

■ HYDROCOLLOID IMPRESSION MATERIAL (REVERSIBLE)

Reversible hydrocolloid is hydrophilic, which means that it adapts to water. It can be used repeatedly by heating and cooling with a unit specially made for this purpose. It is referred to as reversible because it has the capacity to change from a liquid (sol) state to a semisolid (gel) state and back again under specific time and temperature conditions. Due to the costly, specialized equipment needed to heat and house it, reversible hydrocolloid is not commonly used in most practices today. It also requires a special tray set-up which may impede the dentist's chair time. See Table 5-3 for advantages and disadvantages of using this material.

Use

Reversible hydrocolloid impression material is used by the dentist in the fabrication of crown and bridge work and full and partial dentures (not for study models). It is chosen for its high definition in replicating the oral structures.

Mixing Alginate (Irreversible) Impression Material and Loading the Tray

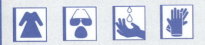

ARMAMENTARIUM

- Alginate bowl and spatula
- Alginate powder
- Alginate powder- (scoop) and water- (cylinder) measuring device
- Impression tray(s)
- Periphery wax
- Topical spray

PROCEDURE

1. Place wax around the periphery of the impression tray, if necessary for patient comfort or to extend the tray.
2. Using the measuring cylinder supplied by the manufacturer, measure the correct amount of room temperature water and pour it into the mixing bowl. Note that the water is always placed in the mixing bowl first. This is to ensure that all of the powder is incorporated correctly into the mixture.
3. Fluff the powder canister, if required by the manufacturer.

4. Fill the measuring scoop by overfilling, then leveling off the top, using the spatula blade perpendicular to the top of the scoop. Dispense the corresponding number of scoops into a second flexible rubber bowl or disposable paper cup.
5. Upon the dentist's direction, pour the powder into the water in the mixing bowl.
6. Mix the water and powder with the stirring motion using the point of the spatula. Then, turn the bowl on its side, holding it securely in the palm of the hand. Rotate the bowl and continue mixing using the widest part of the spatula in a wiping motion around the inside of the bowl (Figure 5-4). Mixing time for Type I alginate takes 45 seconds; for Type II alginate 60 seconds. (Note that mixing time and working time are not the same.)
7. As soon as the mix is homogenous, gather the alginate material onto the spatula and load it into the impression tray (Figure 5-5). Note that on the mandibular tray the material is always loaded from the lingual aspect, in an overlapping technique. This is to help prevent air bubbles from forming in the final model. Use the flat

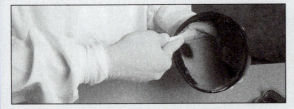

Figure 5-4 The dental assistant mixes the alginate in a flexible bowl using the spatula against the inside of the bowl to spatulate out air bubbles.

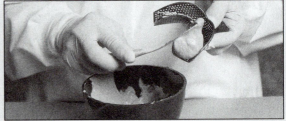

Figure 5-5 The dental assistant loads alginate into a mandibular tray, from the lingual aspect.

of the spatula blade to firmly press the alginate into the tray. When the alginate material is loaded into the tray, moisten a gloved finger with water and lightly smear water along the occlusal portion to help ease insertion into the dental tissues. The tray is now ready to be inserted into the mandibular portion of the oral cavity to take a full-arch impression.

Special Considerations

- Always wear PPE when working at chairside.
- Maintain and work in a clean, dry, aseptic field.
- Clean and disinfect the work area at the conclusion of the procedure, after dismissing the patient.
- Always follow OSHA regulations and CDC recommendations to help prevent the spread of bloodborne diseases and to protect dental personnel.

PRACTICE MAKES PERFECT PROCEDURE ▪ 5-2

Taking an Alginate (Irreversible) Impression

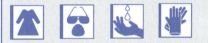

Note: This is a continuation of the previous Practice Makes Perfect Procedure (5-1), Mixing Alginate (Irreversible) Impression Material and Loading the Tray

ARMAMENTARIUM

- Alginate bowl and spatula
- Alginate powder
- Alginate powder- (scoop) and water- (cylinder) measuring device
- Impression tray(s)
- Periphery wax
- Topical spray

PROCEDURE

1. Facing the patient, slightly retract the right cheek. Note that the patient should be seated in an upright position to reduce the likelihood of excess alginate material running down the back of the throat or from being inhaled.

2. Use a small amount of excess alginate from the mixing bowl and using a gloved hand, smear it along the occlusal surface of the mandibular teeth; place extra material in the oral vestibule areas.
3. Invert the tray, making the impression material parallel to the mandibular arch.
4. Turn the tray slightly to facilitate its passing through the opening of the mouth, with one side of the tray entering the oral cavity first, then the other. Use the other hand to retract the lips.
5. When the tray is completely centered in the patient's mouth, center it above the teeth.
6. Lower the tray gently but firmly on the mandibular teeth, placing the posterior area first, then pressing anteriorly.
7. Ask the patient to raise his or her tongue up through the empty space in the middle of the tray and then to move the tongue slightly from side to side.
8. Gently pull out the lower lip from the center using the opposing hand.

9. Complete placing the tray, pushing slightly toward the posterior. This ensures the material will go all the way down into the patient's anterior vestibule to produce an anatomically esthetic, usable model. Leave the tray in a slightly anterior manner by pushing the tray toward the posterior and making certain the lip is out of the way.

10. Allow the mandibular lip to cover the tray, in a relaxed state; it should be close to the handle portion of the tray.

11. Using the index and middle fingers, hold the tray in the patient's mouth (Figure 5-6) until the final set is achieved. Speaking in a calm voice, using an assuring tone, will help the patient to relax. Ask the patient to lower his or her chin to help prevent the material from running down the throat.

12. To check periodically for the final set, press excess material from around the tray periphery or in the bowl. Upon set, the material should feel firm and not change shape when pushed or pinched. When the final set has been achieved, follow Practice Makes Perfect Procedure 5-3: Removing an Alginate Impression for removal from the oral cavity.

13. When taking a maxillary impression, follow steps outlined in Practice Makes Perfect Procedure 5-1: Mixing Alginate (Irreversible) Impression Material and Loading the Tray using powder and water increments for the maxillary arch. Load the maxillary tray from the posterior, in an overlapping technique, to prevent formation of air bubbles, which would distort the final model (Figure 5-7A).

14. Smooth the material using gloved fingers dipped in water (Figure 5-7B). Remove a small amount of impression material from the hard-palate area to prevent excess from going down the back of the patient's throat or from being accidentally aspirated (Figure 5-7C). Smear a small amount of excess alginate onto the occlusal surfaces of the maxillary teeth.

15. Approaching the patient from behind, insert the maxillary tray into the patient's mouth by rotating the tray slightly to facilitate passing it into the oral cavity. Use the other hand to retract the opposite corner of the mouth (Figure 5-7D). Raise the tray to the maxillary arch and retract the lip prior to seating the tray (Figure 5-7E).

16. Instruct the patient to tip his or her head down slightly (this is to reduce the likelihood of gagging) and to breathe through his or her nose until the impression tray is removed. Upon final set, follow the steps in Practice Makes Perfect Procedure 5-3 for removing the impression tray.

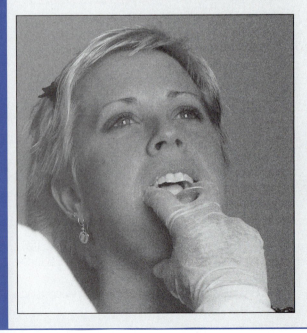

Figure 5-6 The dental assistant holds the mandibular tray in the patient's mouth until the final set is achieved.

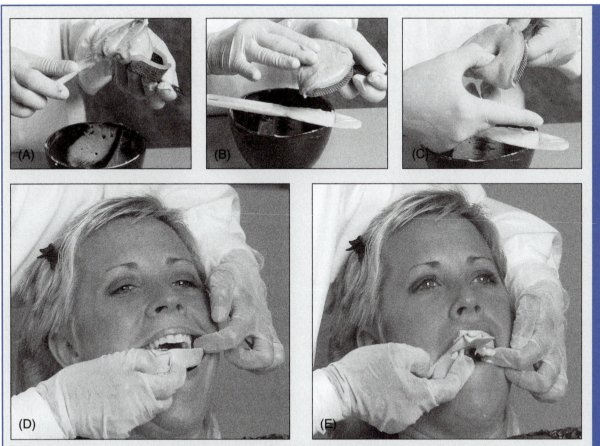

Figure 5-7(A) The dental assistant loads the maxillary tray from the posterior in an overlapping technique to prevent air bubbles. (B) The dental assistant smooths the alginate using wet gloved fingers to facilitate placement. (C) The dental assistant removes a small amount of alginate from the hard-palate portion of the tray to prevent gagging or accidental aspiration of the material. (D) The operator inserts the tray into the patient's oral cavity, one side at a time, then rotates the tray into the mouth. (E) The dental assistant holds the maxillary tray in position until the final set has been achieved.

Special Considerations

- Have the patient tip the head down and breathe through his or her nose when taking maxillary impressions.
- Have patients who tend to gag rinse with cold water prior to the procedure or spray the patient's hard and soft palate with topical anesthetic.
- Have the patient lower his or her chin when taking the mandibular impression to prevent the impression material from running down the throat.
- Always wear PPE when working at chairside.
- Maintain and work in a clean, dry, aseptic field.
- Clean and disinfect the work area at the conclusion of the procedure, after dismissing the patient.
- Always follow OSHA regulations and CDC recommendations to help prevent the spread of bloodborne diseases and to protect dental personnel.

Removing an Alginate Impression

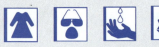

Note: This is a continuation of the previous Practice Makes Perfect Procedures (5-1, 5-2), including the armamentarium.

PROCEDURE

1. After reaching the final set, remove the respective alginate impression tray from the patient's mouth by first loosening the soft tissue of the lips and cheek from around the periphery with the fingers to break the seal.
2. Place the fingers of the opposing hand on the patient's opposite arch to protect the adjacent arch as the tray is being removed.
3. Remove the tray with a gentle but firm snapping motion of the wrist, upward or downward (depending upon the arch). Turn the tray to the side slightly to facilitate removal from the oral cavity.
4. Remove any excess alginate from the patient's mouth with the oral evacuator and have the patient rinse his or her mouth. Check the patient's face for excess alginate. Offer the patient a tissue or moist towelette and a hand mirror to facilitate removal of the material.
5. The dentist will want to examine the impression for accuracy (Figure 5-8).
6. Gently rinse the impression with water to remove visible saliva, blood, or other visible bioburden.

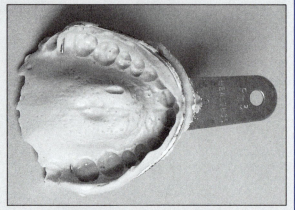

Figure 5-8 The dentist checks the alginate impression for accuracy and detail after removal from the patient's oral cavity.

7. Spray the rinsed impression with an EPA-approved surface disinfectant.
8. If the impression cannot be poured soon, due to time constraints, wrap the impression in a moist (not dripping) paper towel and place inside a humidor or sealed plastic lunch bag labeled with the patient's name. Note that leaving the impression in a moisture-rich environment for too long before pouring will result in imbibition, i.e., absorbing additional moisture, which may distort the final model.

Special Considerations

- Always pay close attention to the patient to ensure that all alginate has been removed from the mouth and face.
- Ask patient if he or she would like some mouth rinse to remove any unpleasant taste left by the alginate.
- Always wear PPE when working at chairside.
- Maintain and work in a clean, dry, aseptic field.
- Clean and disinfect the work area at the conclusion of the procedure, after dismissing the patient.
- Always follow OSHA regulations and CDC recommendations to help prevent the spread of bloodborne diseases and to protect dental personnel.

- Accuracy/fine detail of impression
- Easy manipulation of material
- Allows multiple impressions at a time
- Reusable
- Clean and highly controlled technique
- Can be used for crown and bridge and denture impressions
- Can be used for both hard- and soft-tissue impressions
- Economical (after initial equipment purchase) because the material can be reused

Disadvantages

- High cost of initial equipment (not widely used because of this factor)
- Longer preparation and setting time (10 minutes)
- May lose accuracy due to atmospheric conditions

Table 5-3 Hydrocolloid Reversible Impression Material: Advantages and Disadvantages

Hydrocolloid reversible impression material is supplied by the manufacturer in a solid state; the system employs a combination of injection syringe and water-cooled trays (Figure 5-9).

The tray material is supplied in tubes of five varying viscosities and colors. The specific type used is in accordance with the dentist's preference(s).

The hydrocolloid syringe material is manufactured in three viscosities and forms (stick, back-loading tubes, and preloaded cartridges). The syringe material is also supplied in a variety of colors that denote the respective viscosities. The difference in color between the tray and syringe material provides the dentist and dental laboratory technician with contrast and detail in the final impression.

The system requires the use of a special conditioning unit (Figure 5-10).

Composition

The composition of reversible hydrocolloid impression material is agar-agar (seaweed), water, borax, potassium sulfate, and fillers.

Agar-agar is extracted from seaweed, which provides a suitable base. A colloid provides a suspension of particles (small groups of molecules) in a dispensing medium, in this case water.

Borax is added, in small amounts, to increase the strength of the gel. Borax acts as a retarder

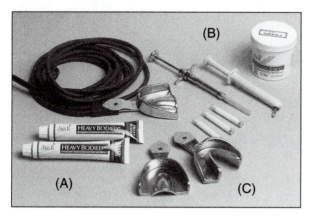

Figure 5-9 Hydrocolloid reversible impression material includes (A) waterline tubes that connect from the tray to the dental unit used to cool the tray material; (B) syringes and cartridges; (C) trays used with the hydrocolloid conditioning to obtain final dental impressions.

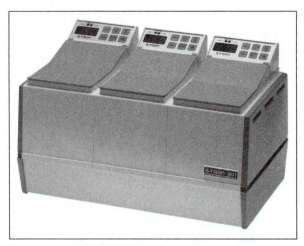

Figure 5-10 B-TRON hydroprocessor.
(Courtesy of Dux Dental.)

for gypsum products to set. Potassium sulfate is added to harden the surface of the stone used in the final pour to provide a more satisfactory finished model. Fillers, flavorings, and preservatives are the remaining ingredients of reversible hydrocolloid impression material.

Properties

Hydrocolloid gels contain relatively weak elastic solids that are subject to tearing easily if stress is applied. After a complete uniform gel is attained, the impression is removed using a quick snapping action.

Gelation of hydrocolloid reversible impression material occurs when cool water [60–70°F (16–21°C)] is circulated through the impression tray from the dental unit via special water tubing connected to the tray for a minimum of 5 minutes.

Hydrocolloid reversible impression material features a number of advantages and disadvantages (see Table 5-3).

Mixing/Manipulation

Hydrocolloid material does not require mixing, as the material is supplied in a variety of tubes and syringe-ready systems. However, first the material must be liquified in the boiling compartment followed by placement in the storage compartments and finally into the tempering compartment of the conditioning unit. The dental assistant moves these tubes or cartridges from these three compartments, from left to right (see Table 5-4).

■ ELASTOMERIC IMPRESSION MATERIALS

Elastomeric impression materials are secondary, more highly detailed impressions than hydrocolloids. Elastomerics are so named because of their rubberlike qualities. Elastomerics are not affected by atmospheric changes; they are more elastic and rubberlike when set, a quality that facilitates their removal from the oral cavity with little or no distortion or tearing.

The three major types of elastomeric impression materials are polysulfide, silicone

Process	Temperatures
Boiling compartment	212°F or 100°C
Storage compartment	150–155°F (66–68°C)
Tempering compartment	110–120°F (43–46°C)

Table 5-4 Hydrocolloid Conditioning

(polysiloxane and polyvinyl siloxanes), and polyether. Each of these has a catalyst and base that are mixed by the chairside dental assistant to form an elastomeric material through a process called **polymerization**.

■ POLYSULFIDE ELASTOMERIC IMPRESSION MATERIAL

Polysulfide impression materials have existed in dentistry for some time; they are often referred to as mercaptan or **rubber-base** impression materials. These materials are classified according to the viscosity (see Table 5-5).

Use

Polysulfide impression material is used for crown and bridge, inlay, and onlay construction. Sometimes it is used for full or partial denture construction. Thus, it can be used for single- or multiple-tooth preparations, quadrants, or full-arch impressions.

Composition

Polysulfide impression material is a two-paste system. The base contains mercaptan polymer (meaning it contains many parts); the accelerator contains lead dioxide, sulfur (which accounts for the characteristic "rotten-egg" smell), and fillers to form a paste. Lead dioxide is the ingredient that gives the final impression its brown color. If the reactor is an organic peroxide, dyes may be added that give it other colors.

Properties

For the properties characteristic of polysulfide impression materials, see Table 5-6.

Mixing/Manipulation

Polysulfide products are dispensed by the manufacturers as a two-paste system. These two pastes are expressed in equal lengths, parallel to each other (but not touching), on a specially provided paper mixing pad and then mixed together using a large laboratory spatula (Figure 5-11).

Two sets of rubber-base mixes are generally spatulated: The heavy-body material is mixed and loaded into a custom acrylic tray. The

---

DID YOU KNOW?

As with all dental materials, polysulfide products must be from the same manufacturer and made specifically to be mixed together. The dental assistant should never attempt to combine materials from different manufacturers.

Type	Use
Very high viscosity	Custom trays
High viscosity	Custom trays
Medium/regular viscosity	Full-arch impressions
Low viscosity/syringe	Used in a specialty syringe expressed around the prepared tooth or teeth to obtain fine detail

Table 5-5 Four Classes of Elastomeric Impression Materials

Composition	Advantages	Disadvantages	Product Examples and Manufacturers
Mercaptan polymer	More working time	Must be poured within 30 minutes	Permlastic (Kerr)
Lead dioxide	High accuracy	Shrinkage	Coe-Flex (Coe)
Sulfur fillers	Great detail Tear-resistant Long shelf life	Difficult to spatulate Relatively long setting time (8–10 minutes)	Omniflex (Coe) Neoplex (Heraeus Kulzer)
Stains clothing		Sulfur-like odor (rotten eggs) Color lacks esthetics	

Table 5-6 Properties of Polysulfide Impression Material

interior surface of the tray must first have been coated with special adhesive to retain the rubber base in the tray when it is being removed from the oral cavity (see Chapter 8: Dental Resins on how to fabricate a custom tray).

The light-body rubber-base mix is begun first, upon the direction of the dentist, and is loaded into a syringe. Note that in some offices two people mix the rubber-base material, concurrently starting with the light-body, then beginning the heavy-body mix as the first assistant loads the light-body material into the syringe. This gives the dentist more working time.

The light-body material is loaded into the rubber-base syringe using quick, repetitious strokes (Figure 5-12). Just before passing the loaded syringe to the dentist the dental assistant expresses a small amount of the material onto the paper mixing pad to ensure that the material flows properly and that the syringe and tip are not clogged (Figure 5-13).

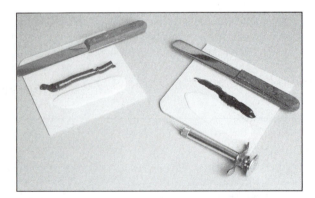

Figure 5-11 Polysulfide impression material is dispensed on paper mixing pads. The dental assistant will note that while the lengths of material are of equal length the amount of the material differs.

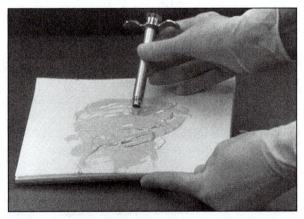

Figure 5-12 The light-body material is loaded into the rubber-base syringe using quick, repetitious strokes.

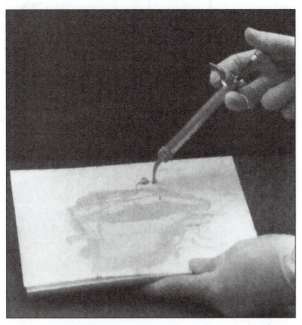

Figure 5-13 The dental assistant expresses a small amount of light-body syringe material onto the paper mixing pad to ensure the flow.

The dental assistant loads the syringe and passes it to the dentist, who expresses the material directly around the prepared tooth or teeth and other oral tissues where fine detail is required. The dental assistant immediately begins mixing the heavy-body material and then loads it into the custom tray and passes it to the dentist.

Whether mixing light- or heavy-body rubber-base impression material, the technique is the same. The dental assistant uses the tip of the laboratory spatula to pick up the accelerator and initially "stir" it into the base (Figure 5-14). This is to initially incorporate the two pastes all the way through to the paper surface of the mixing pad.

The dental assistant continues to mix the rubber-base material, switching to the flat of the spatula blade, making broad, sweeping (stropping) strokes in a figure-8 motion.

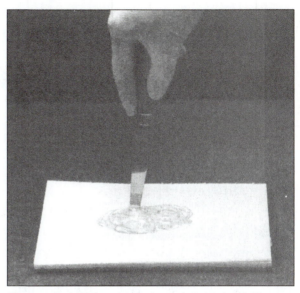

Figure 5-14 The dental assistant initially mixes the rubber-base material by using the point of the laboratory spatula to mix the accelerator into the base.

This is to ensure that there are no air bubbles in the mix and that a homogenous mix results with no white streaks remaining (Figure 5-15).

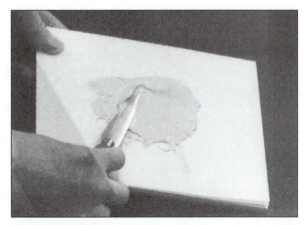

Figure 5-15 The dental assistant uses the length of the spatula to make broad sweeping (stropping) strokes in a figure-8 motion.

Taking a Polysulfide (Rubber-Base) Two-Step Impression

ARMAMENTARIUM

- Mouth mirror, explorer, cotton pliers
- 2 × 2 gauze sponges
- Two tapered laboratory spatulas (tapered)
- Two paper mixing pads supplied by the manufacturer
- Two tubes each of base and accelerator polysulfide impression material
- Rubber-base injection syringe with plastic tip (assembled) and plunger (removed from the syringe)
- Custom tray painted with dried tray adhesive
- Orange solvent
- Syringe brush

PROCEDURE

1. Extrude two sets of rubber-base material (one each of heavy and light body) onto the two respective paper mixing pads. Generally, 4 inches of material is sufficient. If more material is required, additional lines of material can be extruded next to each other on the paper mixing pads.

2. Use 2 × 2 gauze sponges to wipe the mouth of the respective tubes before replacing the caps. (Do not mix accelerator and base 2 × 2 gauzes—take a fresh one to prevent accidental acceleration.)

3. Upon the signal of the dentist, begin mixing the light-body rubber-base material. This is done by using the point of the laboratory spatula to pick up (scrape along the pad) accelerator and stirring it into the base using the point of the spatula.

4. Continue to mix the light-body material with broad, figure-8 stropping motions using the flat of the spatula blade to remove all white streaks to form a homogenous mix. Mixing should be completed within 45–60 seconds.

5. When completely mixed, load the light-body material into the syringe using the back portion of the work-ing end nozzle of the barrel and pushing the syringe over the material repeatedly to force the material into the syringe chamber. Wipe the edges of the syringe with a fresh 2 × 2 gauze sponge. Quickly insert the plunger into the cylinder of the syringe and extrude a small amount onto the end of the mixing pad to ensure proper flow with no clogging.

6. Pass the rubber-base syringe to the dentist with the working end of the syringe pointed toward the arch or quadrant being treated.

7. Mix the heavy-body (tray) material in the same manner, within 45–60 seconds. When completely mixed, gather up the mass of impression material and load it into the custom tray.

8. Receive the empty rubber-base syringe from the dentist and quickly pass the loaded custom tray to the dentist. The total mixing and working time of both types of rubber-base material should not exceed 4 minutes.

9. The impression tray is held in the mouth until completely set. This usually takes a full 6 minutes. Once the tray is completely seated, the dentist may request the dental assistant to continue to hold the tray gently but securely in the patient's mouth until the final set has been achieved.

10. When completion of the set has been achieved, the dentist removes the impression tray using a quick, snapping motion, examines the final impression for the necessary detail, and hands it to the dental assistant.

11. To clean up, peel the set rubber-base material off the laboratory spatulas and the syringe. The plastic syringe nozzle is used only once and discarded. Use the point of the spatula, in a repetitious, gentle motion, to slice around the edges of the pad to remove the top sheet and dispose of it.

12. Use a 2 × 2 sponge moistened with orange solvent to remove any stubborn retained rubber-base material from the spatulas or syringe. Use the syringe brush to clean out the inside of the syringe cylinder.	13. Before dismissing the patient, the dentist will provide the necessary temporary crown coverage of the prepared teeth and the dental assistant will make sure the patient's face is wiped free of any remaining traces of rubber-base material.

Special Considerations

- Have the patient tip the head down and breathe through his or her nose when taking maxillary impressions.
- Have patients who tend to gag rinse with cold water prior to the procedure or spray the patient's hard and soft palate with topical anesthetic.
- Have the patient lower his or her chin when taking the mandibular impression to prevent the impression material from running down the throat.
- Take care not to let polysulfide impression material touch clothing because it leaves a permanent stain.
- Always wear PPE when working at chairside.
- Maintain and work in a clean, dry, aseptic field.
- Clean and disinfect the work area at the conclusion of the procedure, after dismissing the patient.
- Always follow OSHA regulations and CDC recommendations to help prevent the spread of bloodborne diseases and to protect dental personnel.

■ CONDENSATION SILICONE AND POLYSILOXANE/POLYVINYL ADDITION SILICONE ELASTOMERIC IMPRESSION MATERIAL

Condensation silicone and **polysiloxane/polyvinyl** silicone secondary impression materials provide the advantages of polysulfide(s) without the disadvantages. While they are more expensive than polysulfide, they provide high accuracy, no shrinkage, dimensional stability, and high tear resistance with no objectionable odor or taste. They are easier to spatulate than polysulfides.

Use

Silicones have the same use as polysulfides: for crowns and bridges, inlays and onlays, and full-arch impressions. Polyvinylsiloxanes are used for crowns and for edentulous impressions (in the fabrication of dentures).

Composition

Silicone paste is composed of dimethylsiloxane and silica as a reinforcing agent. The silica is added to control the viscosity of the paste; it helps to reduce shrinkage upon polymerization. The catalyst is tin octoate; the reactor is alkyl silicate.

Silicone catalyst is supplied by the manufacturer as either a liquid or a paste. It is spatulated with the accelerator to form silicone rubber.

Polyvinylsiloxane is also known as addition reaction silicone and is more accurate than the conventional condensation silicone. It is available in a range of viscosities for a variety of uses, including the two-phase or putty-wash technique (a technique in which a putty tray and impression material are used together to make a custom tray prior to tooth preparation). The custom tray is used for the final impression.

Properties

For the properties characteristic of silicone impression materials, see Table 5-7.

Mixing/Manipulation

Mixing and manipulation of condensation silicone material is the same as polysulfide impression material. Both materials are expressed in double lines on paper mixing pads and mixed using a laboratory spatula. The light-body material is spatulated first and loaded into a syringe specially made by the manufacturer for the procedure. The heavy-body material is then spatulated and loaded into a custom tray. (Refer to Practice Makes Perfect 5-4 for directions.)

The polyvinyl putty is supplied in two different colors. Each container of putty features a colored scoop used for the base or the catalyst (Figure 5-16). The scoops should not be interused because this may result in contamination of the material and cause polymerization to begin.

The dental assistant dispenses equal amounts of base and catalyst putties. The dental assistant mixes the putty by kneading it quickly until a homogenous color is attained. Mixing time should take no longer than 30 seconds. The material is then placed in the

DID YOU **KNOW?**

Because latex may adversely affect the set of some polyvinyl materials, vinyl examination gloves or vinyl overgloves should be worn when mixing the putty.

Composition	Advantages	Disadvantages	Product Examples and Manufacturers
Condensation Silicone			
Dimethylsiloxane	Easy to handle	Must be poured	Accoe (GC America)
Silica	High accuracy	within 30 minutes	Examix (GC America)
Tin octoate	Odorless	Poor tear strength	Cuttersil (Heraeus
Alky silicate	Patient acceptance	Shorter shelf life	Kulzer)
	is high		Citricon (Kerr)
Polyvinylsiloxane			
Poly(vinyl) siloxane	Good dimensional	Must not contact latex	Express (3M)
Platinum salt	stability	gloves	Extrude (Kerr)
	Ease of handling	May produce hydrogen	Imprint (3M)
	Odorless	gas on setting that	Reprosil (LD Caulk)
	Available in automix	could affect pouring	Omnisil (Coe
	Stability	the cast	Laboratories)
	Short working time	Shorter spatulation and	President (Coltene)
	High accuracy/detail	working time	Hydrosil (LD Caulk)
			Exaflex (GC
			International)

Table 5-7 Properties of Condensation Silicone and Polyvinylsiloxane Impression Materials

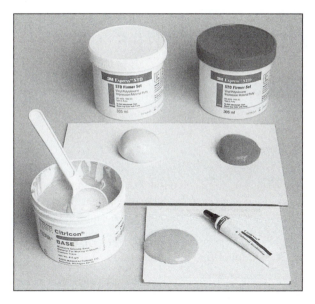

Figure 5-16 Two scoops of putty or putty and a tube of accelerator are dispensed for the putty-wash technique.

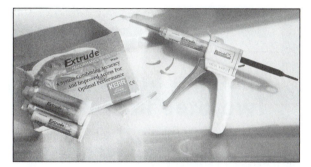

Figure 5-17 Dual-cartridge (automatrix) system used for polyvinylsiloxane impressions.

impression tray. It is then set aside while the dentist prepares the tooth or teeth. This custom tray is used to hold the impression material for the final impression. Final set of the putty material takes about 3 minutes.

With some of the newer polyvinylsiloxane materials a dual-cartridge or automix system is available. With the dual-cartridge system the base paste is in one side of the cartridge and the catalyst paste is in the other (Figure 5-17). When the dentist is ready to take the impression, the putty-wash tray is loaded by squeezing the cartridge-dispensed handle of the extruding hub and engaging the plunger. The plunger then enters the cartridge and extrudes the material through the mixing tip and into the putty material. The dentist can also use the extruding gun to inject the material directly around the sulcus of the prepared tooth or teeth. When ready, the putty tray is placed in the patient's mouth and held until

set. (Fast set takes $3\frac{1}{2}$ minutes; regular set requires 5 minutes.)

After the material has set, the dentist removes the impression using a quick, firm but gently snapping motion, ensuring that the teeth in the opposing arch are protected. The impression is run under cold water and disinfected. Because this material is extremely stable, it is not necessary that it be poured within 30 minutes. In fact, it can be poured weeks later due to its high stability.

In some instances, the dentist may wish to use light-cured silicone impression materials. The setting time is controlled by the operator; however, it is sometimes difficult to move the curing light evenly over the entire surface of the impression material. When using a light-cured impression material, a clear plastic impression tray must be used. The light must penetrate all areas of the impression for curing to result. The curing light acts as a catalyst that brings about polymerization.

■ POLYETHER IMPRESSION MATERIAL

Polyether impression material is fast setting and more accurate than either polysulfide or condensation silicone.

Taking a Silicone (Polysiloxane) Two-Step Impression

ARMAMENTARIUM

- Mouth mirror, explorer, cotton pliers, retraction cord, and retraction placement instrument
- Vinyl exam gloves or vinyl overgloves
- 2 × 2 gauze sponges
- Spatula
- Paper mixing pad supplied by the manufacturer
- Two scoops of the putty, one base and one catalyst, or one putty base and a liquid dropper of catalyst
- Impression tray
- Thin plastic spacer sheet
- Automatrix unit with light-body material
- Dual-cartridge impression material for the automatrix unit
- Mixing tip
- Paper towels

PROCEDURE

Part 1: Preliminary Putty Impression

Note: This portion is completed after the patient has received topical anesthetic injection and prior to tooth preparation.

1. Don vinyl gloves or overgloves.
2. Mix the putty, employing either equal scoops of putty or putty base and drops of catalyst. Knead the putty together until a homogenous mix is achieved. Total optimal time is 30 seconds.
3. Fashion the putty material into a patty and load it securely into the prepared tray. Use the index finger to make a slight indentation or trough to accommodate the area where the teeth to receive the impression are located in the corresponding arch.
4. Place a plastic spacer sheet over the putty material and pass it to the dentist for insertion into the patient's mouth. Setting should be completed in 3 minutes.

5. When the putty portion of the impression has completely set, it is removed from the patient's mouth and the spacer material is removed. The dentist checks the putty impression for accuracy and detail.

Part 2: Automatrix Final Impression

1. After the teeth have been prepared, the area to be replicated is thoroughly cleaned and dried, retraction cord is placed, and the dentist instructs the dental assistant to prepare the final impression (automatrix) material.

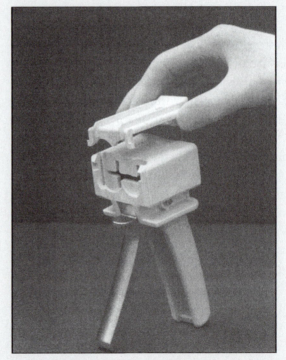

Figure 5-18 The dental assistant assembles the automatrix unit and removes the retainer plate.

2. Prepare the final impression material by loading and preparing the automatrix unit. Remove the retainer plate (Figure 5-18).
3. Insert the plunger by pushing up on the release lever (Figure 5-19).
4. Insert the dual cartridge into the guide grooves on the unit (Figure 5-20).
5. Replace the retainer plate (Figure 5-21). Next, gently squeeze the handle until the plunger makes contact with the cartridge.
6. Remove the protective cap and seal from the cartridge (Figure 5-22).

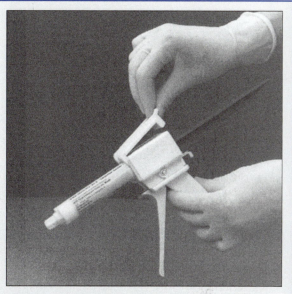

Figure 5-21 The dental assistant replaces the retainer plate.

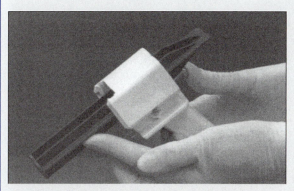

Figure 5-19 The dental assistant inserts the plunger.

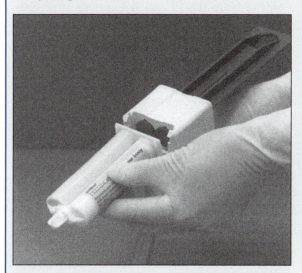

Figure 5-20 The dental assistant inserts the dual cartridge.

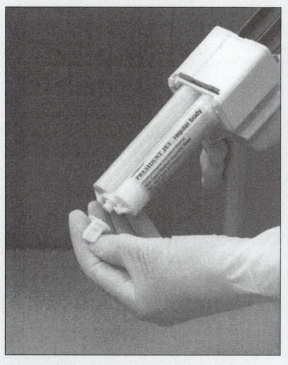

Figure 5-22 The dental assistant removes the protective cap from the cartridge.

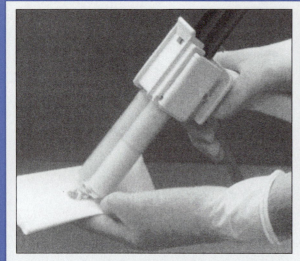

Figure 5-23 The dental assistant expels a small amount of the material.

7. Check the function of the automatrix unit by expressing a small amount of the material onto a paper towel (Figure 5-23).
8. Wipe the end of the cartridge and insert the mixing tip (Figure 5-24) and lock the tip into position by making a one-quarter turn clockwise.

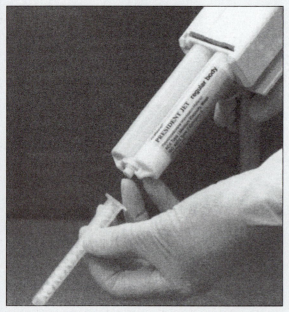

Figure 5-24 The dental assistant inserts the mixing tip.

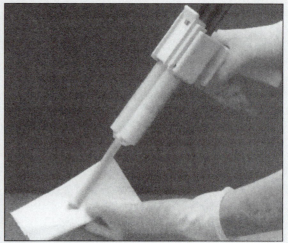

Figure 5-25 The dental assistant tests the flow of the material to ensure impression material delivery is smooth and consistent.

9. Using a firm and continuous pressure, squeeze the handle to test flow of material (Figure 5-25), then expel the desired amount of final impression material into the putty tray directly from the mixing tip (Figure 5-26). Do not remove the mixing tip from the cartridge. (Note that the flow of the material stops when pressure on the handle is released.) The impression material in the mixing tip will set within several minutes. The tip helps seal the cartridge opening, which prevents the impression material from setting. Note that some dentists prefer to inject the automatrix material

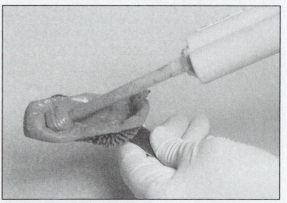

Figure 5-26 The dental assistant extrudes the syringe material from the automatrix syringe into the prepared putty-filled tray.

directly around the prepared teeth, rather than loading it into the putty tray. This procedure is performed according to the individual dentist's preference. In this case, the dental assistant prepares the automatrix unit and then passes it to the dentist, handle first. The dentist uses a continuous application technique to extrude the material directly around the prepared teeth. Next, the dental assistant hands the putty tray to the dentist, who places it over the injected impression material.

10. Hold the tray in place for 5 minutes, allowing the material to set completely.
11. After setting is complete, the dentist removes the impression tray using a firm but gentle quick snapping motion and examines the final impression for detail.
12. The area is cleaned and dried and temporary crowns are applied to the prepared teeth. Prior to dismissing the patient, ensure that all impression material has been removed from the patient's face.

Special Considerations

- Have the patient tip the head down and breathe through his or her nose when taking maxillary impressions.
- Have patients who tend to gag rinse with cold water prior to the procedure or spray the patient's hard and soft palate with topical anesthetic.
- Have the patient lower his or her chin when taking the mandibular impression to prevent the impression material from running down the throat.
- Always wear PPE when working at chairside.
- Maintain and work in a clean, dry, aseptic field.
- Clean and disinfect the work area at the conclusion of the procedure, after dismissing the patient.
- Always follow OSHA regulations and CDC recommendations to help prevent the spread of bloodborne diseases and to protect dental personnel.

Use

Polyether is used for quadrant and full-arch impressions in the fabrication of crowns and bridges. It is supplied in tubes as pastes; the larger tube contains the base, the smaller tube the catalyst. The material is supplied only in regular body, which can be used for both tray material and syringe material. A custom tray prepainted with tray adhesive is used to hold the impression material when taking and removing the impression.

Composition

The base material is a polyether polymer. The catalyst is alky aromatic sulfonate.

Properties

Polyether is easy to manipulate and has less dimensional change during polymerization and storing than polysulfide or condensation silicone impression materials. Because of its high dimensional stability, it need not be poured within the first 30 minutes following setting time.

Because of its hydrophilic nature, polyether should not be exposed to high humidity or stored in water. Because of its overall stiffness, polyether is more difficult to remove from the oral cavity. Care should be taken when working with the catalyst to avoid skin contact, as it may cause skin irritation.

For the properties characteristic of polyether impression materials, see Table 5-8.

Mixing/Manipulation

The polyether impression material is used in a two-step process. The material is dispensed on a paper mixing pad and extruded

Composition	Advantages	Disadvantages	Product Examples and Manufacturers

Polyether polymer
Alky aromatic
  sulfonate
	Easy to handle
	High dimensional
	  stability
	Ease of handling
	No need to pour
	  within 30 minutes
	  after set
	High accuracy/detail
		Must not be stored in
		  humidity or water
		More difficult to remove
		  from the mouth due
		  to stiffness of set
		Catalyst may cause
		  skin irritation
			Impregum (ESPE)
			Permadyne (ESPE)
			Polyjel NF (LD Caulk)

Table 5-8 Properties of Polyether Impression Material

in ribbons of equal length, but not of equal volume (Figure 5-27). Upon the direction of the dentist, the material is spatulated in a stropping or figure-8 motion over a wide area on the mixing pad using a laboratory spatula. The catalyst is lifted using the blade of the spatula and incorporated into the base until a homogenous mixture free of streaks is attained. Mixing should take no longer than 30 seconds.

When spatulation is complete, the dental assistant gathers it onto the spatula and loads it

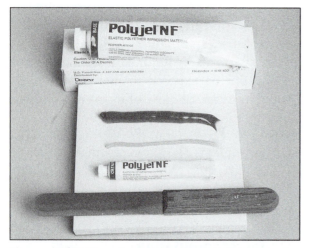

Figure 5-27 The dental assistant dispenses polyether impression material in equal lengths onto a paper mixing pad. A laboratory spatula is used to mix the material.

into the preselected impression tray. It is passed to the dentist, handle first, and placed in the arch or quadrant that will have teeth prepared. In 2 minutes, the dentist agitates the tray slightly to make room for the final polyether impression following preparation of the tooth or teeth. The tray is removed after 3 minutes.

To take the final impression following satisfactory completion of tooth preparation, the dental assistant dispenses the polyether material again, in the same manner. This time, however, less material is needed because the volume of material is already in the preliminary tray.

If the dentist requires a less viscous impression for the syringe portion of the impression, a thinner or body modifier can be added to the mixture.

The dental assistant mixes the catalyst and the modifier into the base material and then loads it into an injection syringe (Figure 5-28). The excess material is loaded into the preliminary impression. The dentist then reinserts the tray into the patient's oral cavity, where it is held by the assistant for 4 minutes to obtain the final impression.

After the final set has been reached, the dentist removes the tray using a gentle but

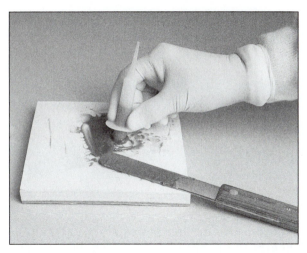

Figure 5-28 The dental assistant back-loads the polyether final impression material into the plastic syringe in a scraping or stropping motion.

firm snapping motion, protecting the opposing arch. The impression is examined by the dentist, rinsed with cold water, and then completely air dried.

After placing temporary crown coverage on the prepared tooth or teeth, the dental assistant makes sure the patient's face is clean of all impression material debris before dismissing the patient.

Spatulation technique for polyether impression material is the same as for polysulfide impression material. Refer to Practice Makes Perfect Procedure 5-4 and follow those steps.

■ DISINFECTION OF DENTAL IMPRESSIONS

The chairside assistant takes an active role in maintaining asepsis of a variety of dental impressions taken in the office. Previously, impressions were allowed to set in the patient's mouth, then rinsed with running water and gently air dried or spray rinsed to remove visible blood and saliva. Today, this is insufficient in reducing the likelihood of infectious disease transmission.

All dental impressions are contaminated with small amounts of the patient's blood and/or saliva and thus carry the potential for cross-infection to other dental team members and to dental laboratory personnel. Some microorganisms may exist for extended periods outside of the human mouth and can be transferred from contaminated impressions to dental cases. If improperly handled, impressions can be a source of cross-contamination.

Impressions are best decontaminated and disinfected (see Table 5-9) at chairside immediately after removal from the oral cavity.

Impression Material	Glutaraldehydes with Phenolic Buffer	Iodophors	Sodium Hypochlorite
Alginate	Recommended	Recommended	Recommended
Polysulfide	Recommended	Recommended	Recommended
Silicone	Recommended	Recommended	Recommended
Polyether	Not recommended	Recommended	Recommended
Reversible hydrocolloids	Not recommended	Recommended	Recommended
Compounds	Not recommended	Recommended	Recommended

Table 5-9 Disinfectants for Dental Impression Materials

Alginate (Irreversible Hydrocolloid) Impressions

Immediately after the impression is removed from the mouth it is rinsed gently under tap water and sprayed with an ADA-recommended disinfectant (Figure 5-29) before it is placed in a zip-locked bag (Figure 5-30). The ADA recommends disinfection of alginate impressions by spraying and wrapping in diluted hypochlorite, iodophor, or glutaraldehyde with phenolic buffer.

Hydrocolloid (Reversible) Impressions

Reversible hydrocolloid impressions may be disinfected by immersion in an iodophor diluted 1 : 213 (5.25 percent), sodium hypochlorite diluted 1 : 10 (2 percent), acid glutaraldehyde diluted 1 : 4, or glutaraldehyde with phenolic buffer diluted 1 : 16.

Polysulfide (Rubber-Base) Impressions

Glutaraldehydes are safe for disinfecting rubber-based impression materials. Because

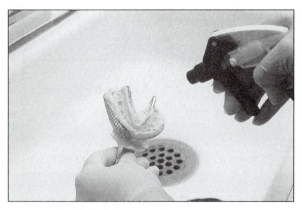

Figure 5-29 The dental assistant sprays the alginate impression with an ADA-approved disinfectant prior to placing it in a zip-locked plastic bag for pouring up later on.

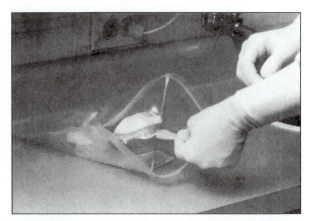

Figure 5-30 The dental assistant carefully inserts the disinfected alginate impression into a plastic zip-locked bag.

some dental impression materials are more sensitive than others and need to be handled using a specific technique or disinfecting solution, it is important that the office have a written policy or procedure that it employs with the commercial dental laboratory.

Elastomeric Impressions

Polysulfides and silicone impression materials are relatively stable and can withstand disinfection without adverse effects by immersion in most disinfectants. Hydrophilic, polyether impressions can also be disinfected by immersion; however, exposure time should be no more than 10 minutes.

Immersion in acid glutaraldehyde has been shown to improve the surface detail reproduction in elastomeric impressions.

■ BITE REGISTRATION

Bite registration is a recording of the patient's normal occlusion when closing the maxillary and mandibular jaws. Bite registration paste is a thin impression or imprint of the occlusal relationship used when the maxillary and mandibular casts are mounted on an articulator.

This bite registration is required by the dental laboratory technician when making a prosthesis or appliance for the patient. Bite registration materials used are either a thin wax wafer with a foil laminate sandwiched in the center of a "U-shaped" wax bite or an impression material of very low viscosity such as heavy-body polyvinylsiloxane silicone. (For wax bite technique, refer to Chapter 7: Dental Waxes.)

When using heavy-body impression material for a bite registration, the material is injected onto the mandibular occlusal/incisal areas of the dentition (Figure 5-31A). The dentist asks the patient to bite down in centric occlusion and the material stays in

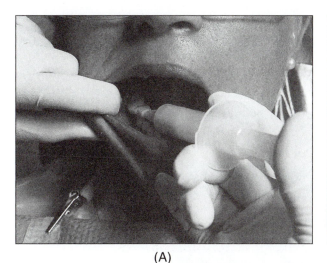

(A)

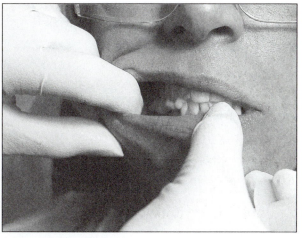

(B)

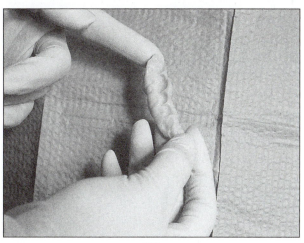

(C)

Figure 5-31 The bite registration material is injected onto the occlusal/incisal areas of the mandibular teeth. The patient closes in centric occlusion. The dentist examines the polymerized bite registration for accuracy and detail.

position until it polymerizes (Figure 5–31B). The dentist then removes the bite registration and examines it for accurately detailed imprints of the teeth in both arches (Figure 5–31C).

■ CRITICAL THINKING QUESTIONS

1. Why are three scoops of alginate powder and three increments of water required for each maxillary full-arch impression, instead of two each as for the mandibular arch?

2. When both maxillary and mandibular impressions are required, the mandibular impression is taken first. Why?

3. What are some of the disadvantages of using polysulfide rubber-base impression material?

4. What are some of the advantages of polyvinylsiloxanes?

5. What is the purpose of taking a bite registration?

Mixing Alginate (Irreversible) Impression Material and Loading the Tray

Student's Name: _____

Date: _____   Instructor: _____

Note: The blank space is provided for the instructor to check off the student's progress. The student may practice the procedure as many times as necessary before being evaluated. Some portions of the exercise may be performed on a typodont, stone tooth model, or extracted tooth or simulated in a clinical operatory. The student has successfully completed the following:

_____ Worn necessary PPE

_____ Assembled necessary armamentarium

_____ Maintained a clear, dry, aseptic working field

_____ Placed wax around the periphery of the impression tray (if necessary) for patient comfort or to extend the tray

_____ Used the measuring cylinder supplied by the manufacturer to measure the correct amount of room temperature water and poured it into the mixing bowl

_____ Fluffed the powder canister, if required by the manufacturer

_____ Filled the measuring scoop by overfilling, then leveled off the top using the spatula blade perpendicular to the top of the scoop

_____ Dispensed the corresponding number of scoops into a second flexible rubber bowl or disposable paper cup

_____ Upon the dentist's direction, poured the powder into the water in the mixing bowl

_____ Mixed the water and power with the stirring motion using the point of the spatula, then turned the bowl on its side, holding it securely in the palm of the hand

_____ Rotated the bowl and continued mixing using the widest part of the spatula in a wiping motion around the inside of the bowl and mixed for the appropriate amount of time (45 seconds for Type I alginate; 60 seconds for Type II alginate)

_____ Gathered the alginate material onto the spatula and loaded it into the respective impression trays

_____ When the material was loaded into the tray, moistened a gloved finger with water and lightly smeared water along the occlusal portion to help easy insertion into the dental tissues

_____ Cleaned and disinfected the work area at the conclusion of the procedure, after dismissing the patient

_____ Followed OSHA regulations and CDC recommendations to help prevent the spread of bloodborne diseases and to protect dental personnel

Comments

_____
_____
_____
_____
_____

PRACTICE MAKES PERFECT
STUDENT ASSESSMENT 5-2

Taking an Alginate (Irreversible) Impression

Student's Name: _____

Date: _____   Instructor: _____

Note: The blank space is provided for the instructor to check off the student's progress. The student may practice the procedure as many times as necessary before being evaluated. Some portions of the exercise may be performed on a typodont, stone tooth model, or extracted tooth or simulated in a clinical operatory. The student has successfully completed the following:

_____ Worn necessary PPE

_____ Assembled necessary armamentarium

_____ Maintained a clear, dry, aseptic working field

_____ Facing the patient, slightly retracted the right cheek (Noted that the patient should be seated in an upright position to reduce the likelihood of excess alginate material running down the back of the throat or from being inhaled)

_____ Used a small amount of excess alginate from the mixing bowl and, using a gloved hand, smeared it along the occlusal surface of the mandibular teeth

When Taking a Mandibular Impression

_____ Inverted the tray, making the impression material parallel to the mandibular arch

_____ Turned the tray slightly to facilitate its passing through the opening of the mouth, with one side of the tray entering the oral cavity first, then the other, and used the other hand to retract the lips

_____ When the tray was completely centered in the patient's mouth, centered it above the teeth

_____ Lowered the tray gently but firmly on the mandibular teeth, placing the posterior area first, then pressing anteriorly

_____ Asked the patient to raise his or her tongue up through the empty space in the middle of the tray and then to move the tongue slightly from side to side

_____ Gently pulled out the lower lip from the center using the opposing hand

_____ Completed placing the tray, pushing slightly toward the posterior

_____ Allowed the mandibular lip to cover the tray in a relaxed state as close to the handle portion of the tray as possible

_____ Used the index and middle fingers to hold the tray in the patient's mouth until the final set was achieved.

_____ Spoke in a calm voice, using assuring tones to help the patient to relax

_____ Checked periodically for the final set by pressing excess material from around the tray periphery or in the bowl

When Taking a Maxillary Impression

_____ Followed steps outlined in Practice Makes Perfect Procedure 5-1 using powder and water increments for the maxillary arch

_____ Loaded the maxillary tray from the posterior, in an overlapping technique, to prevent formation of air bubbles

_____ Smoothed the material using gloved fingers dipped in water

_____ Removed a small amount of impression material from the hard-palate area to prevent excess from going down the back of the patient's throat or from being accidentally aspirated

_____ Smeared a small amount of excess alginate onto the occlusal surfaces of the maxillary teeth

_____ Approached the patient from behind and inserted the maxillary tray into the patient's mouth by rotating the tray slightly to facilitate placing it into the oral cavity

_____ Used the other hand to retract the opposite corner of the mouth

_____ Raised the tray to the maxillary arch and retracted the lip prior to seating the tray

_____ Instructed the patient to tip his or her head down slightly to reduce the likelihood of gagging and to breathe through his or her nose until the impression tray was removed

_____ Cleaned and disinfected the work area at the conclusion of the procedure, after dismissing the patient

_____ Followed OSHA regulations and CDC recommendations to help prevent the spread of bloodborne diseases and to protect dental personnel

Comments

_____

_____

_____

_____

_____

Removing an Alginate Impression

Student's Name: _____

Date: _____   Instructor: _____

Note: The blank space is provided for the instructor to check off the student's progress. The student may practice the procedure as many times as necessary before being evaluated. Some portions of the exercise may be performed on a typodont, stone tooth model, or extracted tooth or simulated in a clinical operatory. The student has successfully completed the following:

_____ Worn necessary PPE

_____ Assembled necessary armamentarium

_____ Maintained a clear, dry, aseptic working field

_____ After reaching the final set, removed the respective alginate impression tray(s) from the patient's mouth by first loosening the soft tissue of the lips and cheek from around the periphery with the fingers to break the seal

_____ Placed the fingers of the opposing hand on the patient's opposite arch to protect the adjacent arch as the tray is being removed

_____ Removed the tray with a gentle but firm snapping motion of the wrist, upward or downward (depending upon the arch), and turned the tray to the side slightly to facilitate removal from the oral cavity

_____ Removed any excess alginate from the patient's mouth with the oral evacuator and had the patient rinse his or her mouth

_____ Checked the patient's face for excess alginate and offered the patient a tissue or moist towelette and a hand mirror to facilitate removal of the material

_____ Gently rinsed the impression with water to remove saliva, blood, or other visible bioburden

_____ Sprayed the rinsed impression with an EPA-approved surface disinfectant

_____ If the impression could not be poured soon, due to time constraints, wrapped the impression in a moist (not dripping) paper towel and placed it inside a humidor or zip-locking plastic bag labeled with the patient's name

_____ Cleaned and disinfected the work area at the conclusion of the procedure, after dismissing the patient

_____ Followed OSHA regulations and CDC recommendations to help prevent the spread of bloodborne diseases and to protect dental personnel

Comments

_____

_____

_____

_____

_____

Taking a Polysulfide (Rubber-Base) Two-Step Impression

Student's Name: _____

Date: _____ Instructor: _____

Note: The blank space is provided for the instructor to check off the student's progress. The student may practice the procedure as many times as necessary before being evaluated. Some portions of the exercise may be performed on a typodont, stone tooth model, or extracted tooth or simulated in a clinical operatory. The student has successfully completed the following:

_____ Worn necessary PPE

_____ Assembled necessary armamentarium

_____ Maintained a clear, dry, aseptic working field

_____ Extruded two lengths of rubber-base material (one each of heavy and light body) onto the two respective paper mixing pads

_____ Used 2 × 2 gauze sponges to wipe the mouth of the respective tubes before replacing the caps

_____ Mixed the light-body rubber-base material by using the point of the laboratory spatula to pick up (scraping along the pad) accelerator and stirred it into the base using the point of the spatula

_____ Continued to mix the light-body material with broad, figure-8 stropping motions, using the flat part of the spatula blade to remove all white streaks to form a homogenous mix within 45–60 seconds

_____ Loaded the light-body material into the syringe using the back portion or the working end nozzle of the barrel and pushed the syringe over the material repeatedly to force the material into the syringe chamber

_____ Wiped the edges of the syringe with a fresh 2 × 2 gauze sponge

_____ Quickly inserted the plunger into the cylinder of the syringe and extruded a small amount onto the end of the mixing pad to ensure adequate flow with no clogging

_____ Passed the rubber-base syringe to the dentist with the working end of the syringe pointed toward the arch or quadrant being treated

_____ Mixed the heavy-body (tray) material in the same manner within 45–60 seconds

_____ When completely mixed, gathered up the mass of impression material and loaded it into the custom tray

_____ Received the empty rubber-base syringe from the dentist and quickly passed the loaded custom tray to the dentist (The total mixing and working time of both types of rubber-base material did not exceed 4 minutes.)

_____ Following final set (6 minutes) and the removal of the impression tray by the dentist, peeled the set rubber-base material off the laboratory spatulas and the syringe; discarded the plastic syringe nozzle; and used the point of the spatula in a repetitious, gentle motion to slice around the edges of the pad to remove the top sheet and disposed of it

_____ Used a 2 × 2 sponge moistened with orange solvent to remove any stubborn retained rubber-base material from the spatulas or syringe

_____ Used the syringe brush to clean out the inside of the syringe cylinder

_____ Made sure the patient's face was wiped free of any remaining traces of rubber-base material

_____ Cleaned and disinfected the work area at the conclusion of the procedure, after dismissing the patient

_____ Followed OSHA regulations and CDC recommendations to help prevent the spread of bloodborne diseases and to protect dental personnel

Comments

_____

_____

_____

_____

_____

PRACTICE MAKES PERFECT
STUDENT ASSESSMENT 5-5

Taking a Silicone (Polysiloxane) Two-Step Impression

Student's Name: _____

Date: _____ Instructor: _____

Note: The blank space is provided for the instructor to check off the student's progress. The student may practice the procedure as many times as necessary before being evaluated. Some portions of the exercise may be performed on a typodont, stone tooth model, or extracted tooth or simulated in a clinical operatory. The student has successfully completed the following:

_____ Worn necessary PPE
_____ Assembled necessary armamentarium
_____ Maintained a clear, dry, aseptic working field

Part 1: Preliminary Putty Impression

_____ Donned vinyl gloves or overgloves
_____ Mixed the putty, using either equal scoops of putty or putty base and drops of catalyst, kneading together until a homogenous mix was achieved (total optimal time 30 seconds)
_____ Fashioned the putty material into a patty and loaded it securely into the prepared tray
_____ Used the index finger to make a slight indentation or trough to accommodate the area where the teeth to receive the impression were located in the corresponding arch
_____ Placed a plastic spacer sheet over the putty material and passed it to the dentist for insertion into the patient's mouth (setting should be completed in 3 minutes)
_____ When the putty portion of the impression had completely set, removed it from the patient's mouth and removed the spacer material

Part 2: Automatrix Final Impression

The dental assistant prepared the final impression material by loading and preparing the automatrix unit using the following steps:
_____ Removed the retainer plate
_____ Inserted the plunger by pushing up on the release lever
_____ Inserted the dual cartridge into the guide grooves on the unit
_____ Replaced the retainer plate
_____ Gently squeezed the handle until the plunger made contact with the cartridge
_____ Removed the protective cap and seal from the cartridge

_____ Checked the function of the automatrix unit by expressing a small amount of the material onto a paper towel

_____ Wiped the end of the cartridge, inserted the mixing tip, and locked the tip into position by making a one-quarter turn clockwise

_____ Using firm and continuous pressure, squeezed the handle to expel the desired amount of final impression material into the putty tray directly from the mixing tip tray

_____ Held the tray in place for 5 minutes, allowing the material to set completely

_____ After setting was complete, removed the impression tray using a firm but gentle quick snapping motion

_____ Cleaned and dried the area and applied temporary coverage to the teeth

_____ Prior to dismissing the patient, ensured that all impression material was removed from the patient's face

_____ Cleaned and disinfected the work area at the conclusion of the procedure, after dismissing the patient

_____ Followed OSHA regulations and CDC recommendations to help prevent the spread of bloodborne diseases and to protect dental personnel

Comments

_____
_____
_____
_____
_____

CHAPTER 5: POSTTEST

Instructions: For each of the following, select the answer that most accurately completes the question or statement.

1. Which of the following fillers are used to make up the bulk of alginate material?
   A. diatomaceous earth
   B. zinc oxide
   C. polysulfide
   D. A and B only
   E. B and C only

2. Alginate impressions are used routinely in dentistry to make upper and lower study models for all of the following *except*
   A. fixed and removable prosthetics
   B. orthodontic appliances
   C. composite restorations
   D. mouth guards and bleaching trays (stents)
   E. provisional restorations and custom acrylic trays

3. Advantages of alginate irreversible impression material include all of the following *except*
   A. ease of mixing and manipulation
   B. economical to use
   C. extremely long working time
   D. meets most accuracy requirements for primary casts
   E. its elastic properties, which allow ease of removal from undercuts found in the oral cavity

4. Working time refers to the time at which the mixed impression material begins to set through a chemical reaction until it is completely set and is ready to be removed from the oral cavity.
   A. True
   B. False

5. When mixing alginate, as the water temperature increases, the working time
   A. decreases
   B. increases
   C. remains unaffected

6. When mixing alginate, which of the following statement(s) is/are true?
   A. Two scoops of powder and two increments of water are required for each mandibular full-arch impression.
   B. Three scoops of powder and three increments of water are required for each maxillary full-arch impression.
   C. The suggested temperature should be room temperature [70°F (21°C)].
   D. All of the above

7. Mixing time for Type I alginate takes _____ seconds.
   A. 45
   B. 60
   C. 90
   D. 120

8. The dental assistant should load the maxillary tray with alginate from the anterior in an overlapping technique to prevent formation of air bubbles, which would distort the final model.
   A. True
   B. False

9. When removing any type of impression tray from the oral cavity, the operator should place his or her fingers of the opposing hand on the patient's opposite arch to
   A. reduce the likelihood of the patient gagging
   B. reduce the likelihood of the patient aspirating excess impression material
   C. reduce the likelihood of air bubbles forming in the set impression
   D. protect the teeth of the adjacent arch as the tray is being removed

10. All of the following statements are true with regard to hydrocolloid reversible impression material *except*
    A. It can be reused.
    B. The tray material is supplied in tubes of five varying viscosities and colors.
    C. It has the same composition and setting time as polysulfide impression material.
    D. The syringe material is supplied in a variety of colors, which denote the respective viscosities.

11. Gelation of hydrocolloid reversible impression material occurs when cool water [60–70°F (16–21°C)] is circulated through the impression tray from the dental unit via special water tubing connected to the tray for a minimum of _____ minutes.
    A. 2
    B. 3
    C. 5
    D. 10

12. Polysulfide impression material can be used for all of the following *except*
    A. fabrication of crowns and bridges
    B. fabrication of inlays and onlays
    C. fabrication of full or partial dentures
    D. single multiple-tooth preparations, quadrants, or full-arch impressions
    E. A and B only
    F. C and D only
    G. all of the above

13. The dental assistant mixes the rubber-base material using the flat of the spatula blade, making broad, sweeping (stropping) strokes in a figure-8 motion to
    A. ensure that there are no air bubbles in the mix
    B. ensure that a homogenous mix results with no white streaks remaining
    C. accelerate the setting/working time
    D. A and B only
    E. B and C only

14. Which of the following are advantages of condensation and addition silicones?
    A. high accuracy
    B. no shrinkage
    C. high tear resistance and dimensional stability
    D. no objectionable taste or odor
    E. A, B, and C only
    F. all of the above

15. Polyvinyl putty features a colored scoop used for the base or the catalyst. These scoops should not be interused because:
    A. Contamination of the material may result.
    B. Polymerization may begin.
    C. Air bubbles or streaking may result in the final mix.
    D. A and B only
    E. B and C only
    F. All of the above

16. Because latex may adversely affect the set of some polyvinyl impression materials, vinyl examination gloves or vinyl overgloves should be worn when mixing the polyvinyl putty.
    A. True
    B. False

17. Polyether is supplied in tubes as pastes; the smaller tube contains the base, the larger tube the catalyst.
    A. True
    B. False

18. Because of its high dimensional stability, polyether impression material needs to be poured within the first 30 minutes following setting time.
    A. True
    B. False

19. All dental impressions are contaminated with small amounts of the patient's blood and/or saliva and thus carry the potential for cross-infection to other dental team members and to dental laboratory personnel.
    A. True
    B. False

20. Which disinfectants are recommended by the ADA for alginate impressions?
    A. diluted hypochlorite
    B. iodophor
    C. glutaraldehyde with phenolic buffer
    D. A and B only
    E. B and C only
    F. all of the above

Gypsum Materials

Chapter 6 Dental Gypsum Materials

To be systematic, believing that system makes for efficiency.

To know the value of time for both my employer and myself.

To safeguard my health, for good health is necessary for the achievement of a successful career.

DENTAL GYPSUM MATERIALS

LEARNING OBJECTIVES

Upon completion of this chapter the student should be able to:

1. Describe the role of the dental assistant in the use, composition, and properties of plaster and stone (gypsum materials) used in dentistry.

2. Describe the steps required for the dental assistant to pour and trim study models for diagnostic purposes in dentistry.

KEY TERMS

articulate

articulator

calcination

die stone

gypsum

(study) model

plaster (Plaster of Paris)

■ INTRODUCTION

Many different types of **gypsum** materials are used in the dental office. The dental assistant must be familiar with gypsum materials as well as with use, composition, and manipulation. Gypsum materials vary in type of product, use, quality, dimensional accuracy, resistance, variation in detail of the oral structures, water-to-powder ratio, and setting and handling times. They are mined of hard rock (calcium) that is ground into a fine powder and heated. The water is removed from the stone using a process called **calcination**.

Used in the dental office, gypsum products are combined with specific amounts of water to create a slurry mixture (see Table 6-1), which is then poured into an impression of the patient's mouth. The gypsum hardens and is separated from the impression and a positive replicate (model) of the dental arch or specific quadrant or tooth remains.

The **model** (or **study model**) is then trimmed according to the dentist's requirements. Study models are most often used in prosthodontics and orthodontics.

■ PLASTER

Plaster (Plaster of Paris) is a white gypsum product also known as calcium sulfate beta-hemihydrate. It is one of the oldest (and weakest) forms of gypsum used in dental practice. When mixed with water, it rehardens to a dihydrate.

Use

Plaster is used for study models and requires more water than other gypsum products. (This also accounts for its brittleness when

Type	Uses	Powder-to-Water Ratio
Plaster (Plaster of Paris)	Study models Opposing models Mounting casts Repairing casts	Unspecific
Type I impression plaster	Edentulous impressions Prosthodontic construction	60 mL : 100 grams
Type II laboratory or model plaster	Study models Diagnostic casts	50 mL : 100 grams
Type III laboratory stone	Study models Diagnostic casts Models for partial and full dentures	30 mL : 100 grams
Type IV die stone	Dies Models or casts for crown and bridge work	24 mL : 100 grams
Type V high-strength, high-expansion die stone	Dies or casts for crown and bridge work	18–22 mL : 100 grams

Table 6-1 Comparison of Dental Gypsum Products

hardened; it is easily subject to fracture.) Plaster is used for opposing models, in mounting study models and casts, and occasionally for repairing casts.

■ TYPE I: IMPRESSION PLASTER

The primary requirement is that Type I impression plaster be sufficiently thick so that it will not run out of the impression trays as it is inserted into the oral cavity.

Use

Type I impression plaster is used for impressions of the edentulous mouth and for certain prosthetic construction procedures. It is mixed with a water-to-powder ratio of 60 mL of water to 100 grams of powder. After placement in the oral cavity, the operator waits for it to set (4–5 minutes) and then gently removes it. It must then be reassembled in the dental laboratory due to its high rate of fracture upon removal from the mouth.

Because better products are available on the market, this material is rarely used for impressions. Instead, it is used primarily to mount casts on articulators because of its quick setting time.

■ TYPE II: LABORATORY OR MODEL PLASTER

Type II laboratory or model plaster is a high-grade plaster, excellent for study models and general work; this is mainly because of its durability and ease of mixing.

Use

Model plaster is most often used by the dental assistant to pour diagnostic casts, also referred to as study models. It is somewhat denser (stronger) than Type I impression plaster. The water-to-powder ratio is 50 mL of water to 100 grams of powder.

■ TYPE III: LABORATORY STONE

Type III laboratory stone is a hard, accurate stone. This high-strength stone has a smooth consistency which provides excellent reproduction of detail for dentists and prosthodontists.

Use

Type III laboratory stone is stronger than plaster and is used where the dentist or prosthodontist requires greater strength. It is used for working casts and for models for partial and full dentures. The dental assistant uses 30 mL of water to 100 grams of powder to mix Type III laboratory stone.

Laboratory stone is most often yellow, due to the pigments added by the manufacturer; it is referred to as calcium sulfur alpha-hemihydrate.

■ ORTHODONTIC STONE

Aside from Type III laboratory stone, Type IV die stone, and Type V high-strength stone, another stone that is commonly used in dentistry today is the orthodontic stone.

Use

Orthodontic stone (as the name implies) is used by orthodontic practices for diagnosis, treatment planning, and case presentation. It is most often white and may be polished for presentation purposes.

TYPE IV: DIE STONE

Type IV **die stone** is calcinated by autoclaving with calcium chloride. This is a modified alpha–hemihydrate. (A die is a positive replica of a prepared tooth for an inlay, onlay, or full crown made from stone.) Because it is denser, it requires even less water for mixing with the powder: 24 mL : 100 grams.

The more stone, the less water, the stronger the final model, with less likelihood of air bubbles or susceptibility to fracture. Type IV die stone is most often used for dies or when a stone model or cast is required.

TYPE V: HIGH-STRENGTH, HIGH-EXPANSION DIE STONE

The newest gypsum material added to the ADA material list is Type V. It requires 18–22 mL of water to 100 grams of water. Currently, it is the strongest (densest) gypsum product available for use in dentistry.

POURING AN ALGINATE IMPRESSION FOR A STUDY MODEL

Prior to pouring an alginate impression in laboratory gypsum or stone, the dental assistant must be familiar with the set and spatulation technique required (Figure 6-1).

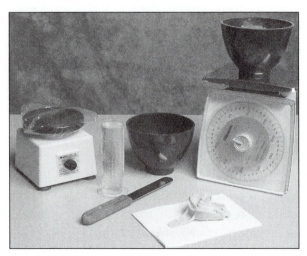

Figure 6-1 Laboratory equipment required by the dental assistant to pour a plaster model.

The setting times of stone and plaster are called initial set and final set. The initial set occurs between the spatulation and the time the mixture loses its gloss and becomes firm or solid enough to handle but is still moist and pliable.

The final set occurs after the plaster of stone has completed crystallization, when all of the heat (exothermic reaction) has been released. At this stage, the stone or plaster is very hard and almost dry. The strength of gypsum increases quickly as the material hardens after the initial set.

Gypsum also has two strengths: wet and dry. Wet strength is present when the water is in excess of that required to bring the gypsum back to its natural water content. After the excess water content has been released or the model or cast has dried, the strength is referred to as dry. The dry strength may be two or more times the wet strength. Box 6-1 lists factors that affect the setting time of gypsum.

In general, the longer the water and gypsum powder are spatulated, the faster the set will

- Refinement (done during manufacturing)
- Water temperature and humidity of atmosphere
- Time and speed of spatulation (mechanical vs. manual)
- Powder-to-water ratio
- Retarders (borax), accelerators (potassium sulfate), or other ingredients added during manufacture

Box 6-1 Factors That Affect Setting Time of Gypsum

take place. The amount of spatulation refers to the time and speed of spatulation. Some offices and dental laboratories spatulate by hand; others use mechanical mixers.

■ SEPARATING, TRIMMING, AND FINISHING DIAGNOSTIC CASTS (STUDY MODELS)

Diagnostic casts (study models) are used to make treatment plan case presentations to patients; they are also used for secondary impressions for crown and bridge and implant procedures. They become a part of the patient's clinical records; they also reflect on the clinical expertise of the office.

PRACTICE MAKES PERFECT PROCEDURE ■ 6-1

Pouring an Alginate Impression: Two-Pour Method

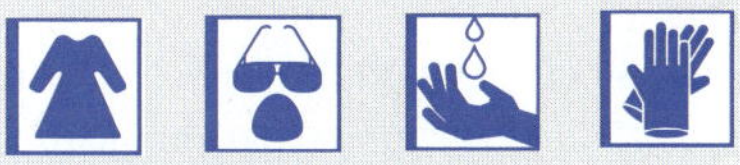

ARMAMENTARIUM
- Metal (narrow) laboratory spatula
- Two flexible rubber mixing bowls
- Gram measuring scale
- 100 grams of plaster
- Calibrated syringe or vial water-measuring device, room-temperature water
- Laboratory vibrator with plastic cover on platform or paper towel
- Alginate impression (disinfected)
- Glass slab or paper towel
- Laboratory knife

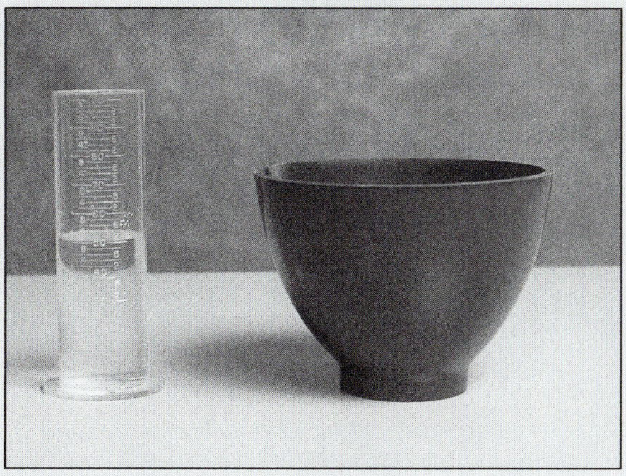

PROCEDURE
Preparing the Gypsum

1. Measure 50 mL of room-temperature water into one of the flexible mixing bowls (Figure 6-2).

Figure 6-2 Calibrated water measure and flexible laboratory mixing bowl. (Bowls for mixing alginate and plaster or stone should be designated as such and not interchanged.)

2. Place the other mixing bowl on the scale; set the dial back to zero. (This allows the dental assistant to weigh the plaster out accurately, without having to adjust for the weight of the bowl.) (See Figure 6-3.)
3. Add the powder from the second bowl into the first bowl of water. Place the water in first to allow for all of the powder to become incorporated into the final slurry mixture. Wait several seconds for the plaster powder to dissolve into the room-temperature water.
4. Using the laboratory spatula, slowly mix the plaster particles together (20 seconds); total mixing time is 60 seconds. (Be sure to mix until all plaster particles are incorporated into the water.)

Pouring the Impression

5. Turn on the laboratory vibrator to medium or slow speed; place the rubber bowl with the slurry plaster mixture on the platform; apply light pressure on the bowl.

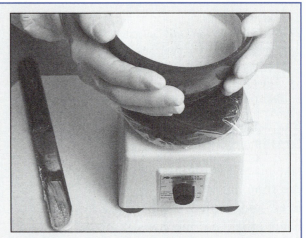

Figure 6-4 The dental assistant uses a laboratory vibrator to bring air bubbles to the surface of the plaster mixture.

6. Rotate the bowl on the vibrator platform; this allows air bubbles to rise to the surface (Figure 6-4). Air bubbles left in the mixture create voids in the final model. Continue mixing and vibrating for 1–2 minutes. (The dental assistant should avoid overvibrating the mixture, as this actually causes additional air bubbles to form.)
7. When the spatula can cut through the mixture and it stays to the sides without moving, the plaster mixture is ready to pour into the impression (Figure 6-5). It will exhibit an appearance of heavy whipped cream.

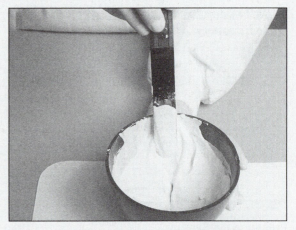

Figure 6-5 The plaster is ready to pour when the mixture retains its position as the spatula is drawn through it.

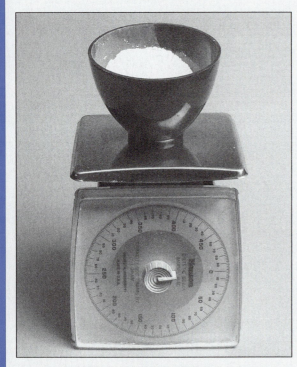

Figure 6-3 The dental assistant measures out 100 grams of plaster to pour the alginate impression.

8. When pouring a mandibular alginate impression, place the impression with tray on the laboratory vibrator and begin loading the plaster mix from either side of the posterior end of the impression (Figure 6-6). When pouring a maxillary impression, begin at the postdam area. Continue to add small increments, each time placing the tip of the spatula into the last increment (from the same side), so as to avoid creating air bubbles or voids in the final model. Complete filling the impression, filling all the areas of the arch, all the way to the opposite end of the impression.

9. After the tooth portion of the impression has been filled completely, place additional plaster, in larger increments, to fill up the entire impression. Set aside for several minutes.

Creating the Base

10. Wipe the rubber bowl and spatula with a paper towel and dispose of the remaining gypsum material. Wash, clean, and ready the rubber bowl and spatula for a second mixture and pour of plaster.

11. The ratio can be changed to 40 mL of water to 100 grams of powder to create a thicker (denser) base. If pouring the base for only one model, use half this amount.

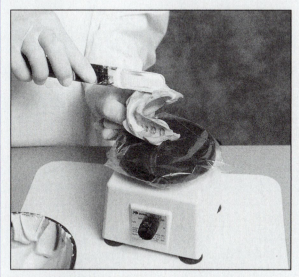

Figure 6-6 The dental assistant pours a mandibular impression, adding small quantities of gypsum to the alginate until the impression is filled.

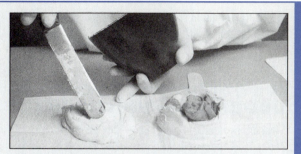

Figure 6-7 The dental assistant gathers a mass of second-pour gypsum (to form the base of the model) on the end of the laboratory spatula and places it on a paper towel (or glass slab). It must be sufficiently dense so as to not flatten out.

12. Mix and vibrate the plaster into the water as outlined previously in steps 4 and 5. The mix will be thicker.

13. Gather up the plaster on the end of the spatula and place it on the glass slab or a paper towel (Figure 6-7). The gypsum mix should have sufficient body to allow it to mass upward and not spread out.

14. After the base pour is on the paper towel or glass slab, invert the poured impression with tray onto the base gypsum material. Hold the tray steady and position the handle so that it is parallel to the paper towel or glass slab surface. This is to ensure that the base is even and uniform. Note that this saves trimming time later and also makes a more esthetically pleasing final model.

15. Finally, carefully drag the excess plaster up over the edges of the cast, filling in any voids (Figure 6-8). The

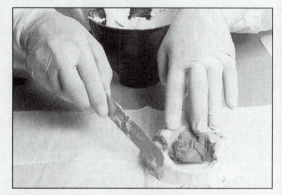

Figure 6-8 The dental assistant smooths out the plaster sides of the base after the impression has been inverted onto it.

dental assistant should avoid covering any margins of the periphery of the impression tray as this will lock the plaster into the tray, making it difficult to separate after the final set.

Special Considerations

- Measure powder and water carefully and mix thoroughly, incorporating all of the powder particles into the water.
- Avoid under- or overvibrating, as this will cause air bubbles to form in the cast(s).
- Do not pour excess slurry down the drain without a specialty trap (to avoid clogging the drainpipes).
- Always wear PPE when working in the laboratory.
- Maintain and work in a clean, dry, aseptic field.
- Clean and disinfect the work area at the conclusion of the procedure.
- Always follow OSHA regulations and CDC recommendations to help prevent the spread of bloodborne diseases and to protect dental personnel.

To ensure an esthetically pleasing appearance, study models should be trimmed and articulated. It is the job of the dental assistant to carefully separate the impressions from the stone model, to then trim them on a model trimmer, and sometimes to **articulate** (match the maxillary to the mandibular occlusion) them together. In some cases, the dentist may also require the casts to be placed on a laboratory **articulator** (a mechanical hinge and frame that holds models of the patient's teeth to maintain the occlusion, representing his or her jaws; the hinge replicates the temporomandibular joints to which upper and lower casts of the dental arches may be attached to simulate oral functions).

Approximately two-thirds of the trimmed study model is comprised of the anatomic portion of the cast (Figure 6-9). The anatomic portion includes the teeth, gingiva, oral mucosa, tori, and frenum attachments; it comprises approximately 1 inch in width. The remaining one-third is the base (sometimes referred to as the art portion) of the cast. The dental assistant trims this in a geometric form,

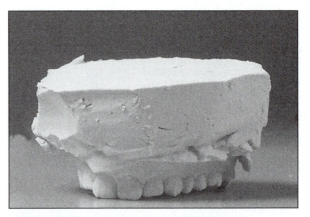

Figure 6-9 An example of how the separated (maxillary) study model appears immediately after separation.

using specific angles. It is about $\frac{1}{2}$ inch wide. When the maxillary and mandibular models are trimmed and in occlusion, their overall height should approximate 3 inches.

To separate the impression from the model, the dental assistant allows approximately 1 hour for the gypsum material to completely set. This is determined by feel:

The exothermic reaction should have completely dissipated. If the plaster is crumbly to the touch, additional setting time should be allowed.

The dental assistant uses a laboratory knife to gently remove any plaster clinging to the margin (periphery) of the tray (Figure 6-10). Holding the handle of the impression tray, the assistant then carefully lifts the tray upward and slightly forward, taking into account the angle of the patient's dentition.

Disinfection of Dental Casts

The dental assistant disinfects dental casts only after the final set has been reached. Stone models should be disinfected with a spray of iodophor used according to the manufacturer's instructions.

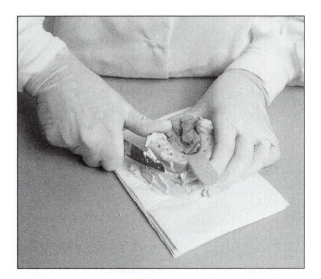

Figure 6-10 The dental assistant uses a laboratory knife to remove excess plaster prior to separating it from the model.

PRACTICE MAKES PERFECT PROCEDURE ■ 6-2

Trimming a Diagnostic Cast (Study Model)

 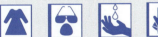

ARMAMENTARIUM
- Maxillary/mandibular models, separated from the impressions
- Two flexible mixing bowls
- Laboratory knife
- Pencil
- Measuring straight edge
- Model trimmer with safety shield and adjustable platform

PROCEDURE
1. Soak the models in water-filled rubber mixing bowls for 5 minutes, prior to trimming. This helps the grinding wheel on the model trimmer to work more efficiently and with less friction.
2. Adjust the water so that it runs freely over the grinding wheel when turned on. (Make sure the sink contains a plaster trap so that excess plaster will not clog the drain.)
3. Invert the models so the teeth rest on the counter. Evaluate the models to determine whether the respective base is parallel to the counter (Figure 6-11).

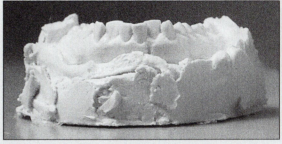

Figure 6-11 The base of the study model should appear parallel to the counter.

4. Switch on the model trimmer and trim the base of each model parallel to the patient's occlusal plane. Use light, even pressure and hold the model securely while trimming (Figure 6-12). Use a back-and-forth motion across the grinding surface.

5. As a safety precaution, rest your wrists on the table of the model trimmer and keep fingers away from the grinding wheel.

6. Place the models together in occlusion to evaluate whether the models are parallel to the counter.

7. When both models are parallel and in occlusion, hold them in occlusion and evaluate which posterior teeth are the most distal. Select that model and use a pencil to draw a line behind the retromolar area (mandibular arch) (Figure 6-13) or postdam area (maxillary arch).

8. Place the base surface of the model on the trimmer table and cut the posterior area at a right angle to the base with the base up to the indicated lines (Figure 6-14).

9. Return the models back into occlusion and place the cut model on the top. Place the opposite base on the model trimmer guide, holding the models together; trim the posterior at a right angle to the base (Figure 6-15). (The trimmed model acts as a guide to follow while trimming the opposing model.)

10. Periodically check to ensure that the backs of the models are trimmed to the same plane by placing

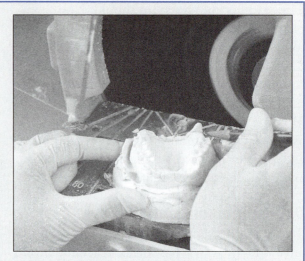

Figure 6-13 The dental assistant uses a pencil to draw a line indicating 2 mm behind the last tooth in the arch on each side.

them, in occlusion, on their backs on a flat surface (Figure 6-16). If the models are kept in occlusion while trimming, the occlusal plane should be at a right angle to the flat surface.

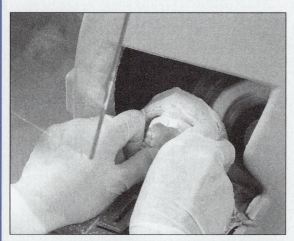

Figure 6-12 The dental assistant holds the study model firmly and maintains even pressure on the grinding wheel of the model trimmer.

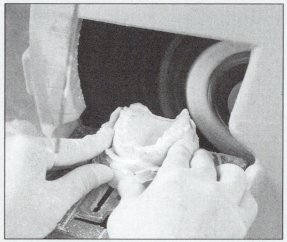

Figure 6-14 The dental assistant follows the pencil markings to trim the posterior base of the model at a right angle to the base.

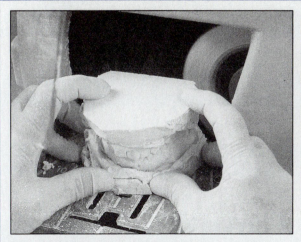

Figure 6-15 The dental assistant places the models back into occlusion and trims the posterior portion.

11. To trim the side angles, use a pencil to mark these areas: outward from the middle of the mandibular premolars to the edge of the model and the maxillary cuspids. Then draw a line running parallel to the teeth at the greatest depth of the buccal vestibules, from the molars to the premolars (about 5 mm from the buccal surface of the teeth). Both models should be marked this way.

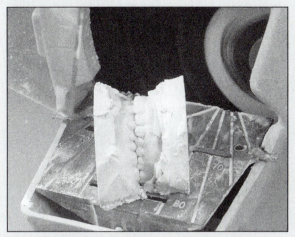

Figure 6-16 The dental assistant places the occluded models on their backs on a flat surface to confirm that the backs are trimmed correctly.

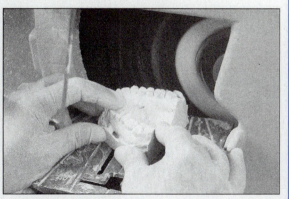

Figure 6-17 The dental assistant trims the vestibule at the deepest area, following the pencil line.

12. Place the model base back on the model trimmer table guide and trim the model to the pencil lines on both sides (Figure 6-17); repeat on the opposing model.
13. Use a pencil dot to mark the midline of the maxillary model in the vestibule area; then use the straight edge of the measure device to draw a line from the dot to the canine on each quadrant (Figure 6-18). Make both of the anterior cuts, forming a point at the midline and center of both cuspids.
14. Mark the mandibular model in a rounded manner from the middle of the canine on one side to the middle of the canine on the opposite side (Figure 6-19).

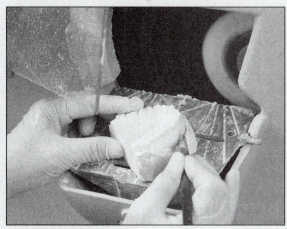

Figure 6-18 The dental assistant draws a line from the midline to the central incisors to the middle of the cuspid to establish an anterior cut line.

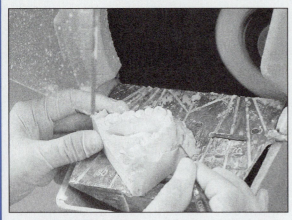

Figure 6-19 The dental assistant draws a rounded line on the mandibular cast from cuspid to cuspid to denote the cut.

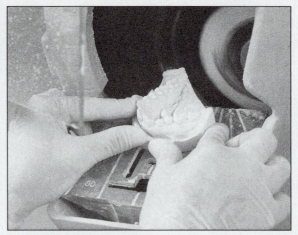

Figure 6-20 The dental assistant makes heel cuts on the models.

15. The heels of both models should be $\frac{3}{8} - \frac{5}{8}$ inches wide and be symmetric in length. The dental assistant can draw on the model by turning the base upward and placing an imaginary diagonal line from the maxillary cuspid to the mandibular premolar to where the side and back cuts meet. Draw a 90° angle across the base, opposite the anterior portion. Heel cuts are small cuts on both models that complete model trimming (Figure 6-20).
16. After the dental assistant has finished trimming the models symmetrically, he or she uses a laboratory knife to trim and smooth the tongue area of the mandibular model.
17. Fill in voids caused by air bubbles with a small amount of plaster.
18. If the dentist prefers, the finished models can be submerged in model gloss for 10 minutes or sprayed with gloss to enhance the esthetic appearance and add strength. The dental assistant then polishes the models using a soft cloth to buff the surfaces for a finished appearance (Figure 6-21).
19. Label both models with the patient's name and the date and place together in a laboratory pan or case box.

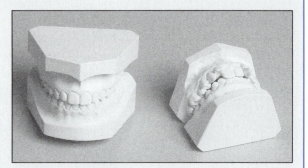

Figure 6-21 The finished trimmed study models take on an esthetically pleasing result.

■ CRITICAL THINKING QUESTIONS

1. Why should the dental assistant place and rotate the bowl on the vibrator platform?
2. Why should the dental assistant avoid covering any margins of the periphery of the impression tray with plaster?
3. Why should the dental assistant soak the models in water-filled rubber mixing bowls for 5 minutes, prior to trimming them?

Special Considerations

- Always soak models prior to trimming.
- Always grasp models prior to trimming.
- Do not allow excess slurry to run down the drain without a specialty trap (to avoid clogging the drainpipes).
- Always label both maxillary and mandibular models with the patient's name and date.
- Always wear PPE when working in the laboratory.
- Maintain and work in a clean, dry, aseptic field.
- Clean and disinfect the work area at the conclusion of the procedure.
- Always follow OSHA regulations and CDC recommendations to help prevent the spread of bloodborne diseases and to protect dental personnel.

PRACTICE MAKES PERFECT
STUDENT ASSESSMENT 6-1

Pouring an Alginate Impression: Two-Pour Method

Student's Name: _____

Date: _____   Instructor: _____

Note: The blank space is provided for the instructor to check off the student's progress. The student may practice the procedure as many times as necessary before being evaluated. Some portions of the exercise may be performed on a typodont, stone tooth model, or extracted tooth or simulated in a clinical operatory. The student has successfully completed the following:

_____ Worn necessary PPE

_____ Assembled necessary armamentarium

_____ Maintained a clear, dry, aseptic working field

Prepared the Gypsum

_____ Measured 50 mL of room-temperature water into one of the flexible mixing bowls

_____ Placed the other mixing bowl on the scale; set the dial back to zero

_____ Added the powder from the second bowl into the first bowl of water; waited several seconds for the plaster powder to dissolve into the room-temperature water

_____ Using the laboratory spatula, slowly mixed the plaster particles together (20 seconds); total mixing time is 60 seconds

Poured the Impression

_____ Turned on the laboratory vibrator to medium or slow speed; placed the rubber bowl with the slurry plaster mixture on the platform; applied light pressure on the bowl

_____ Rotated the bowl on the vibrator platform to allow air bubbles to rise to the surface; continued mixing and vibrating for 1–2 minutes; avoided overvibrating

_____ When the spatula could cut through the mixture and it stayed to the sides without moving, poured the plaster mixture into the impression, exhibiting a heavy whipped cream appearance

_____ When pouring a mandibular alginate impression, placed the impression with tray on the laboratory vibrator and began loading the plaster mix from either side of the posterior end of the impression; when pouring a maxillary impression, began at the postdam area

_____ Continued to add small increments, each time placing the tip of the spatula into the last increment (from the same side), avoiding the creation of air bubbles or voids in the final model

_____ Completed filling the impression, filling all the areas of the arch, all the way to the opposing end of the impression

_____ After the tooth portion of the impression was filled completely, placed additional plaster, in larger increments, to fill up the entire impression; set aside

Created the Base

_____ Wiped the rubber bowl and spatula with a paper towel and disposed of the remaining gypsum material; washed, cleaned, and readied the rubber bowl and spatula for a second mixture and pour of plaster

_____ Mixed a ratio of 40 mL of water to 100 grams of powder to create a thicker (denser) base; if pouring the base for only one model, used half this amount

_____ Mixed and vibrated the plaster into the water as outlined previously

_____ Gathered up the plaster on the end of the spatula and placed it on the glass slab or a paper towel; the gypsum mix had sufficient body to allow it to mass upward without spreading out

_____ After the base pour was on the paper towel or glass slab, inverted the poured impression with tray onto the base gypsum material; held the tray steady and positioned the handle so that it paralleled the paper towel or glass slab surface to ensure that the base was even and uniform

_____ Dragged the excess plaster up over the edges of the cast, filling in any voids

_____ Cleaned and disinfected the work area at the conclusion of the procedure

_____ Followed OSHA regulations and CDC recommendations to help prevent the spread of bloodborne diseases and to protect dental personnel

Comments

_____

_____

_____

_____

_____

PRACTICE MAKES PERFECT
STUDENT ASSESSMENT 6-2

Trimming a Diagnostic Cast (Study Model)

Student's Name: _____

Date: _____   Instructor: _____

Note: The blank space is provided for the instructor to check off the student's progress. The student may practice the procedure as many times as necessary before being evaluated. Some portions of the exercise may be performed on a typodont, stone tooth model, or extracted tooth or simulated in a clinical operatory. The student has successfully completed the following:

- Worn necessary PPE
- Assembled necessary armamentarium
- Maintained a clean, dry, aseptic working field
- Soaked the models in water-filled rubber mixing bowls for 5 minutes
- Adjusted the water so that it ran freely over the grinding wheel
- Inverted the models so the teeth rested on the counter; evaluated the models to determine whether their respective bases were parallel to the counter
- Switched on the model trimmer and trimmed the base of each model parallel to the patient's occlusal plane; used light, even pressure to hold the model securely while trimming with a back-and-forth motion
- Rested his or her wrists on the table of the model trimmer and kept fingers away from the grinding wheel
- Placed the models together in occlusion to evaluate whether they were parallel to the counter
- Used a pencil to draw a line behind the retromolar area (mandibular arch) and postdam area (maxillary arch)
- Placed the base surface of the model on the trimmer table and cut the posterior area at a right angle to the base with the base up to the indicated lines
- Returned the models to occlusion, placing the cut model on the top; placed the opposite base on the model trimmer guide, holding the models together; trimmed the posterior at a right angle to the base
- Periodically checked to ensure that the backs of the models were trimmed to the same plane by placing them, in occlusion, on their backs on a flat surface; ensured the occlusal plane was at a right angle to the flat surface
- To trim the side angles, used a pencil to mark: outward from the middle of the mandibular premolars to the edge of the model and the maxillary cuspids; a line running parallel to the teeth at the greatest depth of the buccal vestibules, from the molars to the premolars (about 5 mm from the buccal surface of the teeth)
- Placed the model base back on the model trimmer table guide and trimmed the model to the pencil lines on both sides; repeated on the opposing model

- Used a pencil dot to mark the midline of the maxillary model in the vestibule area; then used the straight edge of the measure device to draw a line from the dot to the canine on each quadrant; made both of the anterior cuts, forming a point at the midline and center of both cuspids
- Marked the mandibular model in a rounded manner from the middle of the canine on one side to the middle of the canine on the opposite side
- Ensured that the heels of both models were $\frac{3}{8} - \frac{5}{8}$ inches wide and symmetric; drew on the model by turning the base upward and placing an imaginary diagonal line from the maxillary cuspid to the mandibular premolar to where the side and back cuts met; drew a 90° angle across the base, opposite the anterior portion; made small heels on both models
- Used a laboratory knife to trim and smooth the tongue area of the mandibular model
- Filled in voids caused by air bubbles with a small amount of plaster
- Submerged the trimmed models in model gloss for 10 minutes or sprayed with gloss; polished the models using a soft cloth
- Labeled both models with the patient's name and the date and placed together in a laboratory pan or case box
- Cleaned and disinfected the work area at the conclusion of the procedure
- Followed OSHA regulations and CDC recommendations to help prevent the spread of blood-borne diseases and to protect dental personnel

Comments

_____

_____

_____

_____

_____

CHAPTER 6: POSTTEST

Instructions: For each of the following, select the answer that most accurately completes the question or statement.

1. Using a process called calcination, water is added to hard stone to produce gypsum used in dental laboratory procedures.
   A. True
   B. False

2. Study models are most often used in which types of dental procedures?
   A. prosthodontics
   B. orthodontics
   C. endodontics
   D. A and B only
   E. B and C only

3. All of the following are true regarding plaster (Plaster of Paris) *except*
   A. It is a white gypsum product.
   B. It is also known as beta-hemihydrate.
   C. It is one of the newest forms of gypsum approved by the ADA.
   D. It is one of the weakest forms of gypsum used in dentistry.

4. Plaster is used for all of the following applications in dentistry *except*
   A. for opposing models
   B. for mounting study models and casts
   C. occasionally for repairing casts
   D. for taking primary impressions

5. The correct water-to-powder mixing ratio for Type I impression plaster is
   A. 60 mL : 100 grams
   B. 50 mL : 100 grams
   C. 30 mL : 100 grams
   D. 24 mL : 100 grams
   E. 18–22 mL : 100 grams

6. The correct water-to-powder mixing ratio for Type II laboratory or model plaster is
   A. 60 mL : 100 grams
   B. 50 mL : 100 grams
   C. 30 mL : 100 grams
   D. 24 mL : 100 grams
   E. 18–22 mL : 100 grams

7. The correct water-to-powder mixing ratio for Type III laboratory stone is
   A. 60 mL : 100 grams
   B. 50 mL : 100 grams
   C. 30 mL : 100 grams
   D. 24 mL : 100 grams
   E. 18–22 mL : 100 grams

8. The correct water-to-powder mixing ratio for Type IV die stone is
A. 60 mL : 100 grams
B. 50 mL : 100 grams
C. 30 mL : 100 grams
D. 24 mL : 100 grams
E. 18–22 mL : 100 grams

9. The correct water-to-powder mixing ratio for Type V high-strength, high-expansion die stone is
A. 60 mL : 100 grams
B. 50 mL : 100 grams
C. 30 mL : 100 grams
D. 24 mL : 100 grams
E. 18–22 mL : 100 grams

10. The setting time for Type I impression plaster is _____ minutes.
A. 1–2
B. 2–3
C. 4–5
D. 45–60

11. The more stone, the less water, the stronger the final model, with less likelihood of air bubbles or susceptibility to fracture.
A. True
B. False

12. The _____ set of gypsum products occurs between the spatulation and the time the mixture loses its gloss and becomes firm or solid enough to handle but is still moist and pliable.
A. initial
B. final
C. polymerization
D. definitive

13. The _____ set of gypsum products occurs after the plaster or stone has completed crystallization, when all of the heat has been released.
A. initial
B. final
C. polymerization
D. definitive

14. Dry strength of gypsum occurs when the water is in excess of the required amount to bring the gypsum back to its natural water content.
A. True
B. False

15. The total mixing time of laboratory plaster is
A. 10 seconds
B. 20 seconds
C. 30 seconds
D. 60 seconds
E. 2–3 minutes

16. The dental assistant should avoid overvibrating the plaster or stone mixture, as this actually causes additional air bubbles to form.
    A. True
    B. False

17. All of the following statements are true regarding diagnostic casts (study models) *except*
    A. They are used to make treatment plan case presentations to patients.
    B. They are used for secondary impressions for crown and bridge and implant procedures.
    C. They become a part of the patient's clinical records.
    D. They are in no way a reflection of the clinical expertise of the office.

18. When the maxillary and mandibular models are trimmed and in occlusion, their overall height should approximate
    A. 1 inch
    B. 2 inches
    C. 3 inches
    D. 6 inches

19. If the models are kept in occlusion while trimming, the occlusal plane should be at a right angle to the flat surface.
    A. True
    B. False

20. Why should the dental assistant rest his or her wrists on the table of the model trimmer and keep fingers away from the grinding wheel when trimming a model?
    A. to create an esthetically pleasing base for the model
    B. to ensure the correct water-to-powder ratio
    C. to avoid creating hash marks
    D. as a safety precaution

SECTION · V

Related Dental Materials

To be tactful—always doing the right thing at the right time.

To be courteous—for this is the badge of good breeding.

To walk on the sunny side of the street, seeing the beautiful things in life rather than fearing the shadows.

To keep smiling always.

Excerpt from the "Creed for Dental Assistants" by Juliette A. Southard.
Reprinted with the permission of the American Dental Assistants Association, Chicago, IL.

LEARNING OBJECTIVES

Upon completion of this chapter the student should be able to:

1. Describe the general types of waxes used in dentistry and their specific applications.

2. Describe the role and duties of the dental assistant in the care, storage, and handling of dental waxes.

3. Describe specific disinfection procedures as they relate to waxes used in dental procedures.

KEY TERMS

impression (bite registration) wax

pattern wax

processing wax

study wax

undercut wax

■ INTRODUCTION

Various waxes have been used in dentistry for more than 200 years. Waxes used in dental offices today are manufactured from a variety of sources, including bees, plants, and minerals.

Dental waxes are categorized into three general groups: **pattern waxes**, **processing waxes**, and **impression (bite registration) waxes**.

Because they are used directly or indirectly in patients' mouths, dental waxes must be of the highest grade and quality to provide consistent results. Due to the low melting point of some dental waxes, great care must be taken by the dental assistant to store them away from excessive heat to prevent melting or distortion.

■ PATTERN WAXES: USES AND PROPERTIES

Pattern wax, sometimes referred to as inlay wax, is manufactured in dark sticks (Figure 7-1A). Pattern wax is used on a die, which is a positive replica of a prepared tooth poured in laboratory (die) stone. For desirable properties of pattern waxes see Box 7-1.

Pattern waxes vary by manufacturer; however, they share the following general properties:
- Hardness
- Toughness
- Resistance to flaking
- Ability to achieve a smooth surface
- Flow at a temperature slightly above that of the oral cavity
- Achieve complete burnout at temperatures above 900°F
- Carve easily without chipping or cracking

Box 7-1 Properties of Pattern Wax

The properties of pattern wax are vital when utilizing the lost-wax technique for casting prosthetic restorations. Lost wax refers to the wax pattern after the wax is enclosed in investment stone and heated to very high temperatures, which causes the wax to vaporize (hence, "lost wax"). This leaves an empty space where the melted metal (usually dental gold) can be invested using centrifugal force.

Baseplate wax (Figure 7-1B) is a hard (brittle) wax that is heated to form the initial base in processing dentures (Figure 7-2).

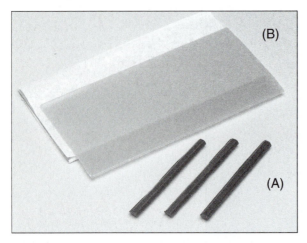

Figure 7-1 Pattern waxes: (A) inlay wax; (B) baseplate wax.

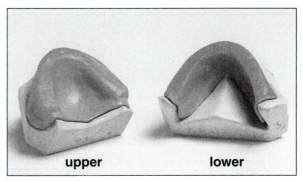

upper   lower

Figure 7-2 Examples of upper (left) and lower (right) baseplates with bite rims processed in the dental laboratory to create full dentures.

■ PROCESSING WAXES

Processing waxes (Figure 7-3) most commonly used in dentistry include boxing wax, utility wax, and sticky wax.

Boxing wax, which is soft and pliable, is used to form a box around an alginate impression prior to pouring it in gypsum. It is supplied in $1\frac{1}{2}$-inch strips and may be reused to make a seal around the impression to hold gypsum in place until the final set.

Sticky wax is very brittle at room temperature; however, when melted with a Bunsen burner or gas flame, it becomes sticky and soft. Sticky wax adheres to many surfaces, including metal, gypsum, and porcelain. An example of a use for sticky wax is to hold two pieces of a broken denture together when making a repair.

Utility wax, often referred to as periphery wax or beading wax, is soft, adhesive, and pliable. It does not require additional heat to be used and it can be molded to most surfaces.

Utility wax is used to bead around the periphery of impression trays to extend them and to facilitate patient comfort. Utility wax is also used by orthodontic patients to cover and cushion brackets and uncomfortable wires until the patient's cheeks and lips heal.

■ IMPRESSION (BITE REGISTRATION) WAXES

Bite registration materials are manufactured as a thin wax wafer with a foil laminate sandwiched in the center of a "U-shaped" wax bite. The purpose of taking a bite registration is to replicate the patient's normal occlusion for the laboratory technician when making a dental prosthesis and in model trimming.

When using the wax wafer to take a bite registration, the wax must be heated in a bowl of warm to hot water to make the wax pliable (bendable). It is then inserted into the oral cavity centered on the mandibular teeth (Figure 7-4A).

The dentist asks the patient to bite down in centric occlusion (normal bite), requiring the patient to place the top of his or her tongue as far back as possible on the palate and to then close. The wax bite remains in that position until the wax has cooled. The dental assistant may be asked to use the air syringe to facilitate cooling of the wax (Figure 7-4B).

The dentist removes the wax bite registration carefully to avoid distortion and observes this impression for sufficient imprints of the occlusal surfaces of the teeth in both arches (Figure 7-4C).

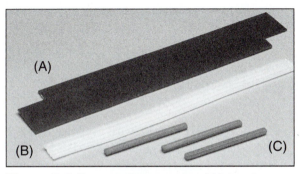

Figure 7-3 Processing waxes: (A) boxing wax; (B) utility wax; (C) sticky wax.

DID YOU **KNOW?**

Inlay wax may also be used to take a bite registration. It is cut to fit the patient's arch and then heated as the wax wafer and inserted into the oral cavity centered on the mandibular teeth.

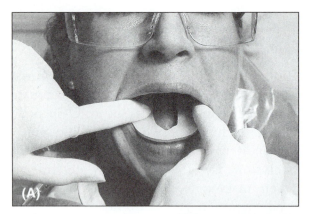
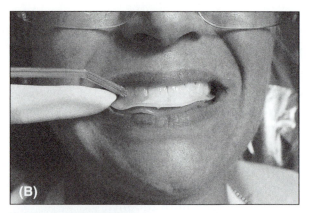
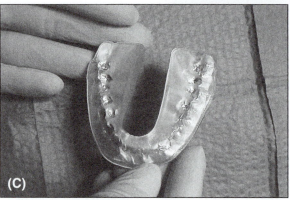

Figure 7-4 (A) When taking a wax bite, the dentist positions the material on the patient's mandibular arch. (B) The dental assistant cools the wax bite using the air syringe. (C) The dentist examines the final wax bite for occlusal detail.

PRACTICE MAKES PERFECT PROCEDURE ▪ 7-1

Taking a Wax Bite Registration

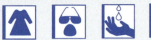

ARMAMENTARIUM
- Basic set-up
- One sheet of bite wax (horseshoe shaped)
- Bowl of warm to hot water
- Air-water syringe

PROCEDURE
1. Place bite wax material into warm to hot water to soften.

2. Remove wax from warm water and place over the patient's mandibular teeth. The bite wax should extend $\frac{1}{4}$ inch beyond the incisal edge of the maxillary central incisors.
3. Ask the patient to close firmly but gently on the wax and to stay closed until the wax has hardened. The patient should be in his or her true centric (closed biting) pattern.
4. Use the air syringe to hasten cooling of the wax.

5. When the wax has cooled completely, carefully remove it and chill it under cold water.
6. Remove the wax from the water and spray it with the appropriate disinfectant.
7. Indicate the patient's initials and the date in the upper right corner of the wax for identification purposes.
8. Before dismissing the patient, ensure that any excess wax has been removed from the patient's lips or face.

Special Considerations

- The wax bite should always remain with the patient's related laboratory case materials, such as study models. Most often, these materials are collected and kept together in a laboratory pan or (case) work pan.
- Always wear PPE when working at chairside.
- Maintain and work in a clean, dry, aseptic field.
- Clean and disinfect the work area at the conclusion of the procedure, after dismissing the patient.
- Always follow OSHA regulations and CDC recommendations to help prevent the spread of bloodborne diseases and to protect dental personnel.

PRACTICE MAKES PERFECT PROCEDURE ■ 7-2

Taking a Bite Registration Using Polysiloxane and Extruder Gun

ARMAMENTARIUM
- Polysiloxane and extruder gun

PROCEDURE
1. Explain to the patient that you will be taking a bite registration.
2. It is always important to practice biting down with your patient. Occasionally the patient has a difficult time positioning his or her teeth in the correct occlusion. In addition, this will allow you to establish the correct occlusion.
3. Instruct the patient to open his or her mouth. Slowly dispense the bite registration material onto the occlusal surface of the lower teeth beginning from right to left to ensure that all occlusal surfaces are covered.
4. Ask the patient to bite together gently, positioning his or her teeth in the correct occlusion. The assistant may assist the patient to ensure proper occlusion.
5. Explain to the patient that the material takes approximately 60 seconds to set. Ask the patient to gently occlude until the material sets.
6. Ask the patient to open and carefully remove the polysiloxane bits.
7. Rinse and disinfect the polysiloxane bite after removal from the mouth. Disinfection with a suitable commercial dental disinfectant solution will not affect the surface or dimension.
8. Place the bite registration in a baggy or container and indicate the patient's name and date.
9. Before dismissing the patient, ensure that any excess material has been removed from the patient's mouth.

Disinfection of Wax Bites

The dental assistant disinfects wax bites using an iodophor recommended by the ADA. For disinfection to be most effective, the item should remain wet with disinfectant for the time recommended for tuberculocidal disinfection (usually 10 minutes).

Wax bites can also be immersed in sodium hypochlorite or sprayed with iodophor.

■ MISCELLANEOUS WAXES

There are other waxes used in dentistry that are not included in the three primary categories. These include **study wax** and **undercut wax**.

Study wax is a hard wax manufactured in blocks. It is used primarily for educational purposes to teach carving of teeth and dental anatomy (Figure 7-5).

Undercut wax is used to fill undercuts of dental structures prior to taking impressions (to prevent the impression material from sticking to the prepared teeth and to facilitate removal of the impression tray).

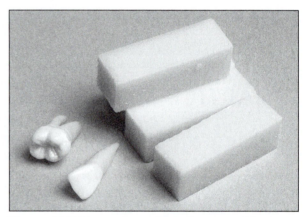

Figure 7-5 Examples of teeth carved in study wax.

■ CRITICAL THINKING QUESTIONS

1. Why must the dental assistant take great care to store dental waxes away from excessive heat?
2. When taking a wax bite, why must the wax bite registration material be heated in a bowl of water first?
3. When taking a wax bite registration, why might the dental assistant be asked to apply compressed air to the wax while the patient holds it in centric position?

PRACTICE MAKES PERFECT
STUDENT ASSESSMENT 7-1

Taking a Wax Bite Registration

Student's Name: _____

Date: _____   Instructor: _____

Note: The blank space is provided for the instructor to check off the student's progress. The student may practice the procedure as many times as necessary before being evaluated. Some portions of the exercise may be performed on a typodont, stone tooth model, or extracted tooth or simulated in a clinical operatory. The student has successfully completed the following:

_____   Worn necessary PPE

_____   Assembled necessary armamentarium

_____   Maintained a clear, dry, aseptic working field

_____   Placed wax bite material into warm to hot water to soften

_____   Removed wax bite material from the warm water and placed it over the occlusal surfaces of the patient's mandibular teeth

_____   Asked the patient to close firmly but gently on the wax and to stay closed until the wax was hardened

_____   Checked to ensure the patient was in his or her true centric (closed biting) pattern when closing down on the wax

_____   Used the air syringe to hasten cooling of the wax bite

_____   When the wax bite was cooled completely, carefully removed it from the patient's mouth and chilled it under cold water

_____   Removed the bite from the water and sprayed it with the appropriate disinfectant

_____   Indicated the patient's initials and the date in the upper right corner of the wax for identification purposes

_____   Before dismissing the patient, ensured that any excess wax was removed from the patient's lips or face

_____   Cleaned and disinfected the work area at the conclusion of the procedure, after dismissing the patient

_____   Followed OSHA regulations and CDC recommendations to help prevent the spread of bloodborne diseases and to protect dental personnel

Comments

_____

_____

_____

_____

_____

Taking a Bite Registration Using Polysiloxane and Extruder Gun

Student's Name: _____

Date: _____   Instructor: _____

Note: The blank space is provided for the instructor to check off the student's progress. The student may practice the procedure as many times as necessary before being evaluated. Some portions of the exercise may be performed on a typodont, stone tooth model, or extracted tooth or simulated in a clinical operatory. The student has successfully completed the following:

_____ Worn necessary PPE

_____ Assembled necessary armamentarium

_____ Maintained a clear, dry, aseptic working field

_____ Explained to the patient that you will be taking a bite registration

_____ Practiced biting down with the patient

_____ Instructed the patient to open his or her mouth

_____ Slowly dispensed the bite registration material onto the occlusal surface of the lower teeth beginning from right to left to ensure that all occlusal surfaces are covered

_____ Asked patient to bite together gently, positioning his or her teeth in the correct occlusion

_____ Assisted the patient to ensure proper occlusion if necessary

_____ Explained to the patient that the material takes approximately 60 seconds to set

_____ Asked the patient to gently occlude until the material sets

_____ Asked the patient to open and carefully remove the polysiloxane bite

_____ Rinsed and disinfected the polysiloxane bite after removal from the mouth

_____ Inserted the bite registration in a baggy or container and indicated the patient's name and date

_____ Before dismissing the patient, ensured that any excess material has been removed from the patient's mouth

_____ Cleaned and disinfected the work area at the conclusion of the procedure, after dismissing the patient

_____ Followed OSHA regulations and CDC recommendations to help prevent the spread of bloodborne diseases and to protect dental personnel

Comments

_____

_____

_____

_____

_____

CHAPTER 7: POSTTEST

Instructions: For each of the following, select the answer that most accurately completes the question or statement.

1. Waxes used in dental offices today are manufactured from a variety of sources, including all of the following *except*
   A. bees
   B. plants
   C. acrylic
   D. minerals

2. All of the following statements are true of pattern wax, *except*
   A. It is sometimes referred to as inlay wax.
   B. It is difficult to carve.
   C. It flows at a temperature slightly above that of the oral cavity.
   D. Achieves complete burnout at temperatures in excess of 900°F.

3. _____ wax is hard and brittle. It is heated to form the initial base in processing dentures.
   A. Processing
   B. Utility
   C. Bite registration
   D. Baseplate

4. Boxing wax is used to
   A. create a tight seal around an alginate impression prior to pouring it in gypsum
   B. ship and box dental crown and bridge cases to send to the outside dental laboratory
   C. create a wax pattern when using the lost-wax technique to make dental prostheses
   D. cover orthodontic bands, wires, or brackets until the patient's lips or cheeks have healed

5. All of the following statements are true regarding sticky wax, *except*
   A. It is brittle at room temperature.
   B. It becomes sticky and soft when heated with a flame.
   C. It is soft and sticky at room temperature.
   D. It adheres easily to many surfaces, including metal, gypsum, and porcelain.

6. _____ wax is used to bead around the periphery of impression trays to extend them to ease patient comfort.
   A. Boxing
   B. Sticky
   C. Bite registration
   D. Utility

7. The purpose of taking a bite registration is to replicate the patient's normal occlusion for the laboratory technician when making a dental prosthesis.
   A. True
   B. False

LEARNING OBJECTIVES

Upon completion of this chapter the student should be able to:

1. Describe the role of the dental assistant in the use, composition, and properties of acrylic and other tray materials used in dentistry.

2. Describe the role of the dental assistant in fabricating temporary (provisional) acrylic restorations.

3. Describe the role of the dental assistant in fabricating self-curing custom resin trays, light-cured custom resin trays, vacuum-formed custom trays, and thermoplastic custom trays.

KEY TERMS

custom tray
flash
matrix
provisional restoration(s)

spacer
thermoplastic reaction
vacuum-formed

■ INTRODUCTION

Resins have been used for many years and have a variety of uses in dentistry. Resins are used not only in restorative procedures; but also to fabricate a variety of **custom trays**. Occasionally, due to our diverse patient population, patients may require a custom tray. The dental assistant may need to fabricate a self-curing custom tray, light-cured custom resin tray, vacuum-formed tray, or a thermoplastic custom tray.

In certain instances the dentist will require a custom tray to be fabricated for a patient (rather than using stock or prefabricated trays).

Use

Regardless of the type of materials used to fabricate it, a custom tray is used in instances where a stock tray will not fit the patient's mouth well or to take a secondary impression for crowns, bridges, and full or partial dentures.

A custom tray may also be used for fabricating a passive (home-administered) tray or stent to hold bleaching solution or gel. A custom tray is fashioned from a stone model of the patient's mouth (Box 8-1).

A custom-fabricated tray should meet or exceed the following criteria:
- Strong enough to hold the material rigid during insertion into and removal from the oral cavity
- Ability to be smoothed and contoured to the dental arch
- Ability to be edentulous, partially edentulous, or full dentition
- Ability to allow for uniform thickness of impression material in all areas of the arch
- Ability to be altered and contoured to fit any irregular area of the arch
- Ability to be designed so that stops are in the spacer to hold the material in stable, specifically designated areas to obtain a highly accurate impression

Box 8-1 Criteria for a Custom Tray

■ RESIN SELF-CURING CUSTOM TRAYS

Custom trays are made from a variety of materials and can be fabricated using self- or light-curing acrylic resin, a vacuum resin, or a thermoplastic material.

The most commonly used material in the fabrication of custom trays is self-curing acrylic tray resin. It has been used for many years in dentistry. Self-curing acrylic tray resin is supplied in a liquid catalyst (monomer) and powder (polymer), which initiates the polymerization process. (Polymerization starts when material changes from a plastic pliable state to a rigid state.)

The initial set occurs when the liquid and powder are mixed together. When pulled apart, it exhibits a "spiderweb" appearance. The second stage takes place when the material can be gathered into a ball, kneaded, and contoured to the dental model. The third stage takes place when the material exhibits an exothermic reaction, giving off a significant amount of heat. The final stage takes place when the heat has diminished and the material is completely rigid. A custom acrylic tray should be fabricated 24 hours prior to use to ensure that stability has occurred.

■ LIGHT-CURED CUSTOM RESIN TRAYS

Acrylic tray resin is also supplied in light-cured custom trays. The main difference between this material and self-curing is that the setting time is controlled by the operator. The material is pliable until a curing light is used to initiate polymerization.

This method requires a special, ovenlike appliance with a special curing light. The custom tray is shaped and placed into the oven for a quick setting; it is then ready for use.

■ VACUUM-FORMED CUSTOM ACRYLIC RESIN TRAYS

A **vacuum-formed** tray is an acrylic tray resin supplied in rigid square sheets that resemble tiles. These sheets are of varying colors and thicknesses (Figure 8-1). The unit has a frame that holds the sheet directly under a heating element (Figure 8-2). When the sheet is softened and it begins to droop (Figure 8-3), the frame drops the sheet onto the cast while vacuum pressure draws and tightly molds and adapts the material to the dental model (Figure 8-4). After allowing sufficient time for the material to cool, the dental assistant removes the vacuum-formed tray from the model and trims it using laboratory scissors (Figure 8-5).

Note that vacuum-formed bleaching stents (trays) and custom orthodontic retainers are

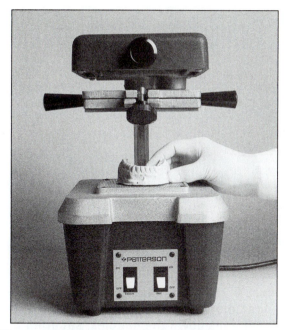

Figure 8-2 The resin sheet is secured in place and the cast is placed on the platform of the vacuum-forming machine. The dental assistant then withdraws his or her hand due to the excess heat generated by the vacuum-forming unit.

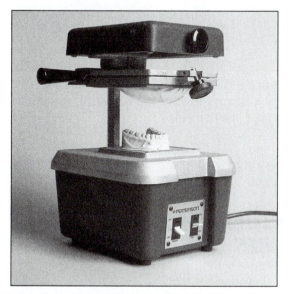

Figure 8-3 Note the resin sheet begins to sag as it is warmed by the heat of the vacuum-forming unit.

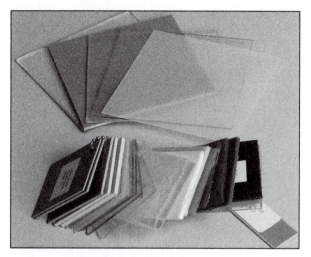

Figure 8-1 Examples of type of vacuum-formed tray/stent materials.

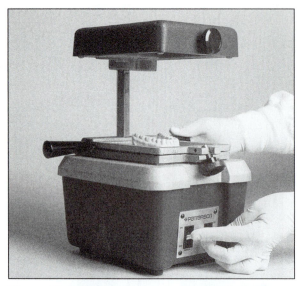

Figure 8-4 When the resin material sags to 1 inch below the holding ring, the dental assistant pulls down the handles, securing the tray material directly over the cast.

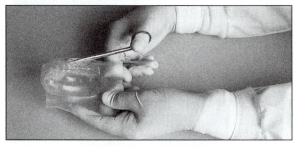

Figure 8-5 The dental assistant uses laboratory scissors to trim the resulting vacuum-formed tray or stent.

fabricated in the same manner but without a handle.

■ THERMOPLASTIC CUSTOM RESIN TRAYS

Thermoplastic beads and buttons are other materials used for fabricating custom trays. A **thermoplastic reaction** takes place when these small, round beads or buttons are placed in warm mater. (Thermoplastic means the material becomes pliable and soft when exposed to heat.)

When the material is softened, the dental assistant conforms it to the dental model into the desired shape. The tray hardens as the heat dissipates.

Mixing and Manipulation of Acrylic Resin Tray Material

Regardless of the type of material used, all custom trays are made using the same principles. It is important for the dental assistant to have an understanding of the necessary preparation prior to making a custom tray.

When making a custom tray for an edentulous model, the dental assistant draws a blue line around the buccal vestibule encompassing the facial periphery and the postdam area (the area at the posterior of the hard palate). This is an outline for the tray material on the maxillary (Figure 8-6).

If fabricating a mandibular tray, the dental assistant draws a horseshoe-shaped blue line around the facial area of the buccal vestibule, continuing around the lingual area, allowing

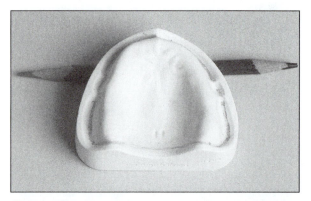

Figure 8-6 The dental assistant outlines the tray margin on the stone cast using a blue pencil, then the area where the spacer is to be placed in red pencil.

room for the patient's tongue to be lifted freely while taking the impression.

The dental assistant then uses a red pencil to mark a second peripheral line 2 mm upward (toward the ridge) of the edentulous model. This red line provides a definitive line to follow when placing a **spacer** on the model to allow room in the tray for the impression material used (or for bleaching solution or gel). The spacer may be made of pink baseplate wax or a commercial nonstick molding material or a moist paper towel.

When the spacer is placed, the dental assistant fills in undercuts to relieve recessed areas in the model that would otherwise prevent the tray from being comfortably placed and removed from the dental arch. Undercuts may be caused by bubbles in plaster, cavities, or the shape of the respective arch or individual teeth. If the dental assistant uses baseplate wax, it must be gently heated using a waving motion of the flame to evenly soften the wax without scorching it; it can be softened in a bowl filled with warm water and adapted to fit the model.

The dental assistant then uses a warm laboratory knife to cut back the spacer material to the red line on the model (Figure 8-7). Next, the dental assistant uses the dental laboratory knife to cut stops in the wax spacer to allow room for the impression material to flow evenly (Figure 8-8).

Self-curing acrylic resin tray material is extremely exothermic. In fact, it heats up

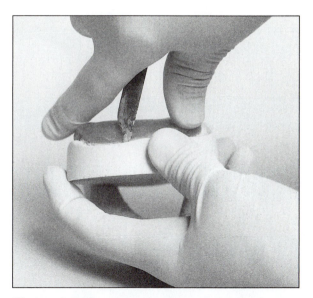

Figure 8-7 The dental assistant trims the pink baseplate wax spacer with a laboratory knife. To avoid slipping or accidental cuts, the dental assistant uses a thumb and forefinger as fulcrum points to steady the model.

sufficiently to cause wax to melt slightly. It may also cause burns or allergic reactions in some people. Thus, the dental assistant should place a sheet of aluminum foil over the wax spacer and into the stops (Figure 8-9). This makes it easier to remove the wax from the tissue side of the tray after the custom tray is fabricated.

After preparing the cast, the dental assistant mixes the acrylic tray resin according to the manufacturer's instructions. While in the doughy stage, the maxillary material can be shaped into a patty and the mandibular tray can be rolled into a log shape prior to placing the material on the respective casts (they are mixed and shaped individually).

The dental assistant then makes and secures a handle for each tray from remaining tray resin material, placing it on the anterior of each respective tray near the midline of the

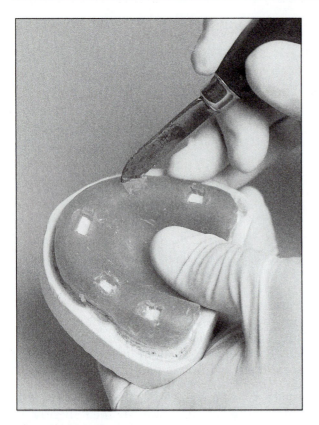

Figure 8-8 The dental assistant uses a laboratory knife to cut stops into the wax spacer. Stops allow room for the impression material to flow properly.

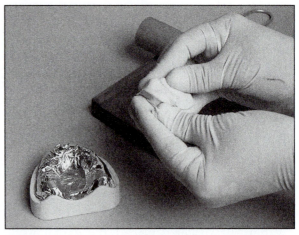

Figure 8-9 The dental assistant kneads the tray resin material and fashions it into a patty, prior to placing it over the edentulous maxillary model. Note the foil in place.

impression, the dental assistant coats the interior of the custom acrylic resin tray with a thin application of adhesive. This keeps the impression material in the tray when removing it from the oral cavity.

Disinfection of a Custom Acrylic Resin Impression Tray

The dental assistant disinfects custom acrylic impression trays by spraying with a surface disinfectant or immersion in either 1 : 213 iodophor or 1 : 10 sodium hypochlorite. The tray should be rinsed thoroughly to remove residual disinfectant, then allowed to dry completely prior to use.

■ CUSTOM PROVISIONAL ACRYLIC RESTORATIONS

In dentistry, the word "provisional" means "serving for the time being" in anticipation of a permanent prosthesis. Whether single-unit crowns or multiple-unit fixed prostheses,

arch. If making a custom athletic mouthguard or passive bleaching tray or stent, no handle is applied. The dental assistant secures the handle by wiping the anterior area of the tray and the handle portion to be attached with resin liquid and then placing the handle on the custom tray and pushing gently. The dental assistant should hold the handle material in a curved fashion until the material has set.

After the final set has taken place, the dental assistant uses an acrylic bur and low-speed handpiece to smooth the peripheral edges of the tray. Prior to taking the secondary

Fabricating a Self-Cured Custom Acrylic Resin Tray

 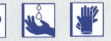

ARMAMENTARIUM

- Maxillary and/or mandibular stone casts
- Red/blue pencil
- Laboratory knife
- Baseplate wax and heat source such as a Bunsen burner or bowl filled with warm water
- Tray resin material: liquid and powder
- Wooden tongue blade and waxed paper cup
- Separating medium with brush, or aluminum foil, or a moist paper towel
- Petroleum jelly
- Tray adhesive

PROCEDURE

Preparing the Cast

1. Outline the cast in blue and red pencil. The red line is drawn 2–3 mm inside the margin of the prepared tooth or teeth or 2–3 mm above the lowest point of the vestibule if the arch is edentulous.
2. Fill in undercuts in the cast; cover with spacer material.
3. Using a laboratory knife, trim the excess wax or spacer material to the red line using an angled cut.
4. Cut stops in the spacer.
5. Cover the spacer with aluminum foil or paint it with separating medium.

Mixing the Self-Curing Acrylic Resin Tray Material

1. Measure the powder and liquid to the correct calibrations on the measuring devices provided by the manufacturer.
2. Spatulate the powder and liquid together with the wooden tongue depressor in the wax paper cup until a homogenous mix is achieved.
3. Allow the mixture to go through the initial polymerization for 2–3 minutes.

4. Apply petroleum jelly to the cast and on the palms of gloved hands.

Contouring the Self-Curing Acrylic Resin Tray Material

1. When the material is no longer sticky, gather it into a ball. Knead it to further mix the materials. Set aside a small amount for a handle.
2. Fashion it into a patty for a maxillary tray or into a log for a mandibular tray.
3. Place the tray material onto the tray and conform it to the arch, extending it to the blue pencil marking or 1–2 mm past the wax spacer (Figure 8-10).
4. Use a laboratory knife to trim back excess material.
5. Use the set-aside material to form a handle. Attach it to the anterior midline by dabbing a small amount of

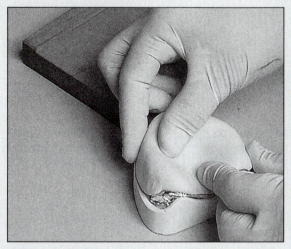

Figure 8-10 The dental assistant carefully adapts the acrylic resin tray material over the wax spacer and aluminum foil on a maxillary cast.

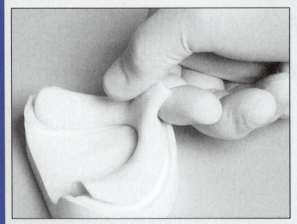

Figure 8-11 The dental assistant attaches the handle to a mandibular custom acrylic resin tray.

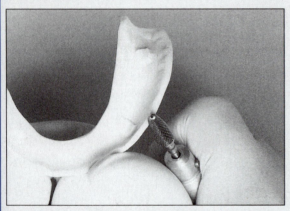

Figure 8-12 The dental assistant uses an acrylic bur and laboratory handpiece to trim the edges of the custom acrylic resin trim after the final set has taken place.

monomer onto the tray and the end of the handle to be attached to the tray. Hold the handle in place to prevent drooping until the material has set (Figure 8-11).

6. After final set (about 30 minutes), use an acrylic bur to smooth excess material from the periphery of the tray. (Do not trim the inside of the tray.) (See Figure 8-12.)

7. Clean and disinfect the tray according to directions that follow.

8. If the dentist is ready to use the custom tray, apply a thin coat of the adhesive inside the custom tray and along the margins (Figure 8-13). Otherwise, return the custom tray to the model and add the patient's name for easy identification.

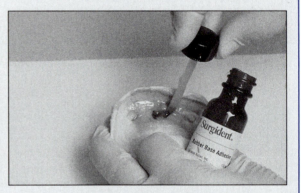

Figure 8-13 The dental assistant paints a thin coat of adhesive to the interior of the tray prior to using it to take an impression. The adhesive holds the impression material in the tray upon removal from the oral cavity.

Special Considerations

- Remember to apply petroleum jelly to the cast and on the palms of gloved hands.
- Avoid breathing fumes released by the tray materials.
- Keep tray materials away from an open flame or matches.
- Allow the heat released from the exothermic reaction to dissipate prior to handling the tray material.
- Always wear PPE when working in the laboratory.
- Maintain and work in a clean, dry, aseptic field.
- Clean and disinfect the work area at the conclusion of the procedure.
- Always follow OSHA regulations and CDC recommendations to help prevent the spread of bloodborne diseases and to protect dental personnel.

Fabricating a Vacuum-Formed Acrylic Resin Custom Tray

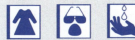

ARMAMENTARIUM

- Casts of maxillary and/or mandibular arches
- Laboratory knife
- Laboratory scissors
- Vacuum-former unit with heating element
- Spacer (if indicated)
- Acrylic sheets (tray material)
- Alcohol torch

PROCEDURE

Preparing the Cast

1. Prior to fabricating the tray(s), soak the cast(s) in warm water for 30 minutes. This helps eliminate small air bubbles from percolating—coming to the surface—between the cast and the acrylic sheet.
2. Place spacer material if necessary. (Baseplate wax is not used with a vacuum former because the extreme heat from the unit would melt the wax.)
3. Use a pencil to mark the desired outer margin (periphery) of the custom tray.
4. Place the cast directly on the center of the vacuum-forming unit.

Contouring the Sheet During Vacuum-Forming Process

1. Select the appropriate acrylic resin sheet(s) from which to fabricate the tray(s).
2. Place the acrylic sheet between the heater frame and the gasket frame and tighten the knob to secure the material in place for warming.

3. Make sure the heating element is in the correct position directly above the acrylic resin sheet.
4. Turn on the heating element. This may take several minutes. The dental assistant should be cautious to avoid touching the cast or platform, as the heat will become intense.
5. Observe the resin as it heats. As it is heated, it will sag. When the resin droops downward approximately 1–2 inches, use both hands on the handles of the frame and pull the frame down, over the cast.
6. Immediately turn on the vacuum after the resin sheet covers the cast entirely.
7. Turn off the heating unit.
8. Allow the vacuum to continue to run for 1–2 minutes to allow the resin to cool until it becomes firm again.

Finishing the Vacuum-Formed Acrylic Resin Custom Tray

1. After the resin has cooled completely, remove it from the vacuum-form frame.
2. Separate the tray from the cast with a laboratory knife.
3. Use laboratory scissors to trim the periphery of the tray to the indicator line.
4. Use an alcohol torch to heat and apply a cutout handle section to the custom tray.
5. Clean and disinfect the tray according to the manufacturer's instructions.
6. Write the patient's name on the model and replace tray on the model, ready for use.

provisional restorations provide many important functions (Box 8-2).

Use

Provisional restorations are used to temporarily provide esthetic, occlusal, and pulpal protection and coverage to a tooth or teeth that have been prepared for a single-unit crown or a multiple-unit bridge. There are two basic types of provisional restorations: direct and indirect. Direct means fabricated directly from the patient's mouth; indirect is fabricated using a stone or gypsum model of the patient's mouth.

Resin custom provisional restorations fitted to the prepared tooth or teeth are one of the better choices for provisional restorations because resin:

- Can be contoured and shaded to meet anatomic, esthetic, and occlusal needs
- Can be made to fit prepared dental margins snugly
- Resists short-term occlusal wear

Composition

The most common types of resin used for provisional restorations are: polymethyl methacrylate, polyethyl methacrylate, and bis-acrylic resin. They each feature a number of advantages and disadvantages (see Table 8-1).

Functions of a Provisional Restoration

- Provides interim treatment that protects the prepared teeth against trauma
- Provides patient comfort
- Maintains function
- Restores appearance

Essentials of a Provisional Restoration

- Soft-tissue health
- Reduced sensitivity of prepared teeth
- Proper occlusion without the necessity of adjusting opposing teeth or new crowns at the time of restoration seating
- Acceptable esthetics while wearing the temporary restoration(s)
- Adequate wound closure of prepared dentin
- Interim phonetics
- Biocentric registration
- Tight final restoration contact areas that resist food impaction or mesial or distal adjacent tooth movement
- Adequate coverage of all prepared surfaces to limit microleakage
- Functional occlusal relationship
- Healthy periodontal environment that can be easily cleaned and maintained by the patient
- Stability of the position of the prepared, adjacent, and opposing teeth
- Protection of the prepared teeth from potential trauma
- Prevention of noxious stimuli from irritating pulpal tissues

Box 8-2 Functions and Essentials of Provisional Restorations

Advantages	Disadvantages
Polymethyl Methacrylate (PMMA)	
• Available in several shades to meet patients' esthetic needs • Relatively easy to mix and manipulate into the crown • Low in cost • Provides high strength and very good color stability over time • Adapts well to the prepared tooth and internal surfaces of the crown • Offers a relatively short setting time • Sufficiently hard to withstand chewing and other functional stresses • Can be trimmed, contoured, and polished easily	• High exothermic properties upon setting • Subject to shrinkage • Potential irritation to the pulp and soft tissues • Localized allergic reaction to the monomer in some patients and dental personnel • Distortion during setting requires adjustments prior to temporarily seating the provisional crown • The resin's limited translucence limits cosmetic quality • Resin easily stains from ingested substances • Difficult to remove if the material sets on the tooth • Leakage may occur unless the margins are well sealed by temporary cement
Polyethyl Methacrylate (PEMA)	
• Low in cost • Provides moderate strength • Provides moderate color stability for several weeks • Provides good adaptation to tooth structures	• Undergoes significant color change if used more than several weeks • Provides inadequate strength for some thin crowns or long-span bridges • Gives off moderate exothermic reaction that requires caution to avoid harm to the dental pulp
Combination Methyl and Ethyl Methacrylate	
• Simple • Adequate provisional restoration • Suitable for multiple-unit restorations • Is a combination of a thin laboratory-manufactured PMMA shell made preoperatively, lined with PEMA in the mouth after the teeth have been prepared. • Is one of the best and least expensive choices where multiple-unit fixed protheses require provisional restorations	• No disadvantages
Bis-acrylic Resin	
• Features a low exothermal reaction • Good adaptation and fit • Moderate color retention • Strength • Safe to use due to lack of exothermic reaction	• Significantly more expensive than PMMA or PEMA

Table 8-1 Advantages and Disadvantages of Provisional Acrylic Materials

Mixing/Manipulation

The following describes the procedure for fabricating a custom acrylic provisional restoration using the direct method. The procedure requires an alginate or silicone putty (primary) impression of the tooth because it will be used as a mold or **matrix** (shape used in dentistry to replicate a natural tooth of the original tooth before it is prepared for a crown). After the preparation has been made by the dentist, acrylic resin is mixed and flowed into the primary impression. When it loses its gloss, the provisional restoration is refitted onto the prepared tooth and left on until the acrylic resin reaches a doughy or rubbery stage.

The impression is then removed and the new provisional restoration takes shape while it polymerizes. It is then gently removed from the prepared tooth without distortion to be trimmed and shaped while taking it on and off the prepared tooth until it reaches the final polymerization.

It must be trimmed to be adapted to the prepared tooth to fit and protect well but so as not to impinge on the gingival tissue or obstruct the interproximal spaces of adjacent teeth. The excess **flash** (extraneous material that extends beyond the cavosurface or gingival margins) must be removed while the resin is still somewhat doughy or rubbery. Finishing discs and sandpaper discs and a polishing agent are used to smooth the finished resin provisional restoration prior to temporary cementation.

PRACTICE MAKES PERFECT PROCEDURE ▪ 8-3

Fabricating an Acrylic Resin Provisional Restoration

ARMAMENTARIUM
- Alginate or silicone putty impression of the tooth or teeth prior to preparation
- Self-curing resin (powder and liquid)
- Dappen dish
- Cement spatula
- Petroleum jelly
- Acrylic/finishing burs and sandpaper discs, mandrel
- Curved crown and bridge scissors
- Polishing agent (prophy paste, prophy cup, contra-angle handpiece)
- Articulating paper with holder
- Temporary cement, paper pad, or automix and applicator instrument
- Dental engine
- Dental floss

PROCEDURE
1. Make an "overimpression" of alginate or silicone putty while awaiting the onset of anesthesia. The impression must include the tooth or teeth to be prepared plus one tooth mesially and distally.
2. Gently rinse the impression and place it in an airtight container such as a locking plastic or vinyl sandwich

bag to keep it moist until after the tooth preparations are made.

3. After tooth preparation is completed, lubricate the prepared tooth or teeth and one tooth adjacent mesially and distally using petroleum jelly (when constructing on a typodont for classroom purposes).

4. Mix the monomer (liquid) and polymer (powder) in a dappen dish using a small spatula; the mix should be sufficiently thick to "trail" 1–2 inches from the spatula.

5. Flow the mix into the original impression. Set it aside until it loses its gloss.

6. Place the impression with the mix onto the prepared tooth or teeth and hold it there until the material reaches a rubber texture or has reached the initial set (2 minutes).

7. Remove the impression from the mouth (typodont) and inspect the new provisional restoration for air voids (bubbles).

8. Carefully work the provisional restoration off the impression, taking care to avoid distortion.

9. Using curved laboratory scissors or a handpiece with acrylic/finishing burs and sandpaper discs, trim the flash while the acrylic resin is still in the rubbery stage. (Figure 8-14)

10. Work the provisional restoration on and off the tooth (typodont) while the material undergoes exothermic reaction and until it attains the final polymerization. Continue trimming the provisional restoration to adapt to the margins of the tooth or teeth.

11. Use a polishing agent to make the provisional restoration smooth and glossy.

12. Use temporary cement to cement the new provisional restoration in place (see Practice Makes Perfect Procedure 3-3: Mixing Zinc Oxide Eugenol Cement (Two-Paste System) in Chapter 3).

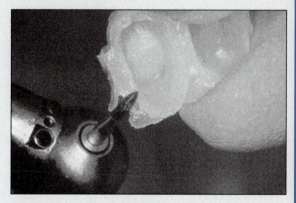

Figure 8-14 Trimming the acrylic resin provisional restoration by removing the flash.

Special Considerations

- Lubricate the prepared tooth or teeth and one tooth adjacent mesially and distally using petroleum jelly.
- Avoid breathing fumes released by the acrylic provisional materials.
- Keep acrylic provisional materials away from an open flame or matches.
- Always wear PPE when working in the laboratory.
- Maintain and work in a clean, dry, aseptic field.
- Clean and disinfect the work area at the conclusion of the procedure.
- Always follow OSHA regulations and CDC recommendations to help prevent the spread of bloodborne diseases and to protect dental personnel.

■ CRITICAL THINKING QUESTIONS

1. Why must the dental assistant avoid handling acrylic resin material during the exothermic stage?

2. Why should the dental assistant be careful not to touch the model or acrylic resin sheet when the heater is turned on in the vacuum–former unit?

3. When fabricating an acrylic resin provisional restoration, why should the dental assistant work the temporary restoration on and off of the typodont?

PRACTICE MAKES PERFECT
STUDENT ASSESSMENT 8-1

Fabricating a Self-Cured Custom Acrylic Resin Tray

Student's Name: _____

Date: _____ Instructor: _____

Note: The blank space is provided for the instructor to check off the student's progress. The student may practice the procedure as many times as necessary before being evaluated. Some portions of the exercise may be performed on a typodont, stone tooth model, or extracted tooth or simulated in a clinical operatory. The student has successfully completed the following:

_____ Worn necessary PPE
_____ Assembled necessary armamentarium
_____ Maintained a clear, dry, aseptic working field

Prepared the Cast

_____ Outlined the cast in blue and red pencil; the red line 2–3 mm inside the margin of the prepared tooth or teeth or 2–3 mm above the lowest point of the vestibule if the arch was edentulous
_____ Filled in undercuts in the cast; covered with spacer material
_____ Using a laboratory knife, trimmed the excess wax or spacer material to the red line using an angled cut
_____ Cut stops in the spacer
_____ Covered the spacer with aluminum foil or painted it with separating medium

Mixed the Self-Curing Acrylic Resin Tray Material

_____ Measured the powder and liquid to the correct calibrations on the measuring devices provided by the manufacturer
_____ Spatulated the powder and liquid together with the wooden tongue depressor in the wax paper cup until a homogenous mix was achieved
_____ Allowed the mixture to go through the initial polymerization for 2–3 minutes
_____ Applied petroleum jelly to the cast and on the palms of gloved hands

Contoured the Self-Curing Acrylic Resin Tray Material

_____ When the material was no longer sticky, gathered it into a ball; kneaded it to further mix the materials; set aside a small amount for a handle
_____ Fashioned it into a patty for a maxillary tray, into a log for a mandibular tray
_____ Placed the tray material onto the tray and conformed it to the arch, extending it to the blue pencil marking or 1–2 mm past the wax spacer

_____ Used a laboratory knife to trim back excess material

_____ Used the set-aside material to form a handle; attached it to the anterior midline by dabbing a small amount of monomer onto the tray and the end of the handle to be attached to the tray; held the handle in place to prevent drooping until the material was set

_____ After final set (about 30 minutes), used an acrylic bur to smooth excess material from the periphery of the tray

_____ Cleaned and disinfected the tray according to directions provided

_____ Returned the tray to the model; added the patient's name for easy identification or, if dentist was ready to use the custom tray, applied a thin coat of the adhesive inside the custom tray and along the margin

_____ Cleaned and disinfected the work area at the conclusion of the procedure

_____ Followed OSHA regulations and CDC recommendations to help prevent the spread of bloodborne diseases and to protect dental personnel

Comments

_____
_____
_____
_____
_____

Fabricating a Vacuum-Formed Acrylic Resin Custom Tray

Student's Name: _____

Date: _____ Instructor: _____

Note: The blank space is provided for the instructor to check off the student's progress. The student may practice the procedure as many times as necessary before being evaluated. Some portions of the exercise may be performed on a typodont, stone tooth model, or extracted tooth or simulated in a clinical operatory. The student has successfully completed the following:

_____ Worn necessary PPE
_____ Assembled necessary armamentarium
_____ Maintained a clear, dry, aseptic working field

Prepared the Cast

_____ Prior to fabricating the tray, soaked the cast in warm water for 30 minutes to help eliminate small air bubbles from percolating
_____ Placed spacer material if necessary
_____ Used a pencil to mark the desired outer margin (periphery) of the custom tray
_____ Placed the cast directly on the center of the vacuum-forming unit

Contoured the Sheet During Vacuum-Forming Process

_____ Selected the appropriate acrylic resin sheet from which to fabricate the tray
_____ Placed the acrylic sheet between the heater frame and the gasket frame and tightened the knob to secure the material in place for warming
_____ Made sure the heating element was in the correct position directly above the acrylic resin sheet
_____ Turned on the heating element
_____ Observed the resin as it heated
_____ When the resin drooped (approximately 1–2 inches) used both hands on the handles of the frame and pulled the frame down, over the cast
_____ Immediately turned on the vacuum after the resin sheet covered the cast entirely
_____ Turned off the heating unit
_____ Allowed the vacuum to continue to run for 1–2 minutes to allow the resin to cool until it became firm again

Finished the Vacuum-Formed Acrylic Resin Custom Tray

_____ After the resin cooled completely, removed it from the vacuum-form frame

_____ Separated the tray from the cast with a laboratory knife

_____ Used laboratory scissors to trim the periphery of the tray to the indicator line

_____ Used an alcohol torch to heat and to apply a cutout handle section to the custom tray

_____ Cleaned and disinfected the tray according to the manufacturer's instructions

_____ Wrote the patient's name on the model and replaced the tray on the model

_____ Cleaned and disinfected the work area at the conclusion of the procedure

_____ Followed OSHA regulations and CDC recommendations to help prevent the spread of bloodborne diseases and to protect dental personnel

Comments

_____

_____

_____

_____

_____

Fabricating an Acrylic Resin Provisional Restoration

Student's Name: _____

Date: _____   Instructor: _____

Note: The blank space is provided for the instructor to check off the student's progress. The student may practice the procedure as many times as necessary before being evaluated. Some portions of the exercise may be performed on a typodont, stone tooth model, or extracted tooth or simulated in a clinical operatory. The student has successfully completed the following:

_____ Worn necessary PPE

_____ Assembled necessary armamentarium

_____ Maintained a clear, dry, aseptic working field

_____ Took an "overimpression" of alginate or silicone putty while awaiting the onset of anesthesia; the impression included the tooth or teeth to be prepared plus one tooth mesially and distally

_____ Gently rinsed the impression and placed it into an airtight container to keep it moist until after the preparations were made

_____ After tooth preparation was completed, lubricated the prepared tooth or teeth and one tooth adjacent mesially and distally using petroleum jelly

_____ Mixed the monomer (liquid) and polymer (powder) in a dappen dish using a small spatula; the mix was sufficiently thick to "trail" 1–2 inches from the spatula

_____ Flowed the mix into the original impression; set it aside until it lost its gloss

_____ Placed the impression with the mix onto the prepared tooth or teeth and held it there until the material reached a rubber texture or reached the initial set (2 minutes)

_____ Removed the impression from the typodont and inspected the new provisional restoration for air voids (bubbles)

_____ Carefully worked the provisional restoration off the impression, taking care to avoid distortion

_____ Used curved laboratory scissors or a handpiece with acrylic/finishing burs and sandpaper discs to trim the excess flash while the acrylic resin was still in the rubbery stage

_____ Worked the provisional restoration on and off the typodont while the material underwent exothermic reaction and until it attained the final polymerization; continued trimming the provisional restoration to adapt to the margins of the tooth or teeth

_____ Used a polishing agent to make the provisional restoration smooth and glossy

_____ Used temporary cement to cement the new provisional restoration in place
_____ Cleaned and disinfected the work area at the conclusion of the procedure
_____ Followed OSHA regulations and CDC recommendations to help prevent the spread of bloodborne diseases and to protect dental personnel

Comments

_____

_____

_____

_____

_____

CHAPTER 8: POSTTEST

Instructions: For each of the following, select the answer that most accurately completes the question or statement.

1. A custom tray may be used for any of the following clinical indications *except*
   A. in instances where a custom or stock tray will not fit the patient's mouth well
   B. to take a secondary impression for crowns, bridges, and full or partial dentures
   C. for orthodontic banding
   D. for fabricating a passive (home-administered) tray or stent to hold bleaching solution or gel

2. A custom-fabricated tray should meet or exceed the following criteria *except*
   A. be strong enough to hold the material rigid during insertion into and removal from the oral cavity
   B. be able to be smoothed and contoured to the dental arch
   C. be adaptable to an edentulous, partially edentulous, or a full dentition
   D. be suitable for taking an alginate (primary) impression in all areas of the arch
   E. be able to be altered and contoured to fit any irregular area of the arch
   F. be able to be designed so that stops are in the spacer to hold the material in a stable, specifically designated area to obtain a highly accurate impression

3. Custom trays are made from a variety of materials and can be fabricated using any or all of the following *except*
   A. spacer
   B. self-curing acrylic resin
   C. light-curing acrylic resin
   D. vacuum resin
   E. thermoplastic material

4. The most commonly used material in the fabrication of custom trays is a
   A. spacer
   B. self-curing acrylic resin
   C. light-curing acrylic resin
   D. vacuum resin
   E. thermoplastic material

5. A vacuum-formed tray is an acrylic tray resin supplied in rigid square sheets of varying colors and thicknesses that resemble tiles.
   A. True
   B. False

6. After allowing sufficient time for the vacuum-formed tray material to cool, the dental assistant removes tray from the model and trims it using
   A. a prophy cup and polishing agent
   B. an acrylic finishing bur
   C. a laboratory scissors
   D. a laboratory knife

7. A thermoplastic reaction takes place when a material becomes pliable and soft when exposed to heat, then returns to its original state when cooled.
   A. True
   B. False

8. What is the purpose of spacer material?
   A. It creates stops.
   B. It allows room in the tray for the impression material or bleaching gel.
   C. It creates an exothermic reaction.
   D. It is used as the secondary impression material for crowns, bridges, and full or partial dentures.

9. The spacer may be made of any or all of the following materials *except*
   A. pink baseplate wax
   B. commercial nonstick molding material
   C. asbestos
   D. a moist paper towel

10. Undercuts may be caused by any or all of the following *except*
    A. bubbles in plaster
    B. cavities
    C. the shape of the respective arch or individual teeth
    D. chewing gum

11. Why does the dental assistant use a combination of fingers and thumbs as fulcrum points?
    A. to work at an even pace
    B. to ensure that his or her gloves are properly worn
    C. to avoid accidental cuts or slipping
    D. to eliminate air bubbles or voids from forming on the tray

12. Prior to taking the secondary impression, why does the dental assistant coat the interior of the custom acrylic resin tray with a thin application of adhesive?
    A. to create a spacer
    B. to keep the impression material in the tray when removing it from the oral cavity
    C. to create an exothermic reaction
    D. to adhere the tray to the stone model

13. Why should the dental assistant hold the handle of the acrylic resin tray in place until the material has set?
    A. to dissipate the heat caused by the exothermic reaction
    B. to facilitate even placement of the impression material
    C. to even the spacer material
    D. to prevent drooping

14. All of the following methods are acceptable for disinfecting a custom acrylic resin impression tray *except*
    A. a sprayed surface disinfectant
    B. immersion in a 1 : 213 iodophor
    C. Lysol
    D. immersion in a 1 : 10 sodium hyopchlorite solution

15. Baseplate wax is an ideal spacer material when using a vacuum former because the heat from the unit evaporates the wax completely.
    A. True
    B. False

16. An ideal provisional restoration should perform all of the following functions *except*
    A. provide interim treatment that protects the prepared tooth or teeth against trauma
    B. provide permanent protection and esthetic appearance of the prepared teeth
    C. provide patient comfort
    D. maintain function
    E. restore appearance

17. The fabrication, placement, and cementation of provisional restorations is essential for which of the following reasons?
    A. soft-tissue health
    B. reduced sensitivity of prepared teeth
    C. acceptable esthetics
    D. adequate wound closure of prepared dentin
    E. all of the above

18. Resin custom provisional restorations fitted to the prepared tooth or teeth are one of the better choices for provisional restorations for all of the following reasons *except*
    A. Resin can be contoured and shaded to meet anatomic, esthetic, and occlusal needs.
    B. Resin can be made to fit prepared dental margins snugly.
    C. Resin closely resembles gold- or silver-colored dental restorations.
    D. Resin resists short-term occlusal wear.

19. What is the purpose of a matrix in dentistry?
    A. It creates a shape used to replicate a natural tooth or the original tooth shape.
    B. It provides room for the impression material.
    C. It eliminates the exothermic reaction.
    D. It serves as a sedative agent to the dental pulp.

20. What does the term "flash" mean in dentistry?
    A. a bright light radiating from the x-ray machine
    B. extraneous material that extends beyond the cavosurface or gingival margins
    C. brightness from the light-cured resin tray material unit
    D. light reflected from the dental treatment room light

PREVENTIVE, BLEACHING, AND SEDATIVE MATERIALS

LEARNING OBJECTIVES

Upon completion of this chapter the student should be able to:

1. Describe the role of the dental assistant in the use, composition, and properties of fluoride(s) in preventive dentistry.

2. Describe the role of the dental assistant in the use, composition, and properties of pit and fissure sealants in preventive dentistry.

3. Describe the role of the dental assistant in the process of tooth bleaching as it relates to cosmetic dentistry.

4. Describe the role of the dental assistant in the use, composition, and properties of periodontal surgical dressings and endodontic sealers and cements.

KEY TERMS

endodontic sealers and
   cements
fluoridation
fluoride

periodontal surgical
   dressing
sealant, pit and fissure
tooth bleaching (whitening)

Important: Some of the procedures described in this chapter may be considered expanded duties, subject to approval of the State Board of Dental Examiners in the respective state of employment. Dental assistants are advised to check their State Dental Practice Act prior to performing these duties on patients.

■ INTRODUCTION

The dental assistant has a variety of duties to perform in the dental office. Each state has a State Board of Dental Examiners with Dental Practice Acts which varies from state to state. Procedures such as applying topical fluoride, pit and fissure sealants, in-office nonvital and vital tooth bleaching, passive tooth bleaching, placement of noneugenol periodontal dressing, and knowledge of endodontic sealers and cements may be considered expanded duties. A dental assistant should check with his or her dentist or the local state board to see which of these duties are permissible in his or her state.

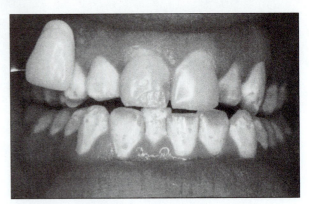

Figure 9-1 Dental fluorosis caused by ingestion of too much systemic fluoride. (One part per million is the recommended optimal level.)

(Courtesy of Dr. Ola Englund.)

■ FLUORIDE

Fluoride has been recognized as a significant factor in the reduction of tooth decay for many decades. Fluoride is a naturally occurring mineral derived from fluorine. **Fluoridation** is the process of optimally adding and adjusting fluoride to the public water supply.

The optimal level of fluoride is one part per million (ppm), that is, one part of fluoride to one million parts of water, delivered in most community/public water systems. Just as too little fluoride is less effective in preventing dental caries, too much fluoride may cause unsightly mottling (Figure 9-1) or dark staining of the enamel. In extreme amounts, fluoride is actually toxic.

Fluoride has also been demonstrated to have a significant therapeutic effect in the control of certain types of periodontal conditions.

Fluoride may be administered two ways: systemically (throughout the body's system) or topically (applied to the site of use).

Systemic Fluoride

When ingested systemically, fluoride works by causing the crystal structure of tooth enamel to be more resistant to acids produced by oral bacteria.

Fluoride is normally ingested through drinking water at a rate of 1 ppm. Fluoride supplements may also be administered from 6 months to age 14 years in liquid or tablet form.

It should also be noted that most bottled or home-filtered drinking water does not contain sufficient fluoride necessary to deliver the optimal level. Thus, parents may wish to add a fluoride supplement to their child's diet, on the recommendation of the dentist and testing of other fluoride levels.

Topical Fluorides

Three types of topical fluoride administered in the dental office are sodium fluoride, stannous fluoride, and acidulated phosphate fluoride (APF). They have varying compositions and applications (Table 9-1).

Type	Composition	Recommended Application	Considerations
Sodium fluoride	2% aqueous	4 times: ages 3,7,10, and 13	Relatively stable Does not stain teeth Has an acceptable taste Does not cause gingival inflammation
Stannous fluoride	8 or 10% aqueous	Every 6 to 12 months	Highly unstable, requiring that a new solution must be dispensed or prepared for each application Unpleasant in taste May stain demineralized areas of enamel, porcelain, or resin restorations May cause sloughing of gingival tissues or gingivitis May aggravate certain existing periodontal conditions
Acidulated phosphate fluoride	1.23% solution, gel, or thixotropic plus 0.1 M orthophosphoric acid	Every 6 months	Easy to use and apply Pleasant flavors available Should not be used with porcelain or composite restorations

Table 9-1 Topical Fluoride Comparison Chart

Sodium Fluoride

Sodium fluoride (or neutral fluoride) is a 2 percent aqueous (water-based) solution administered in a series of four applications. The highest degree of efficacy of sodium fluoride is when it is applied to newly erupted teeth at the ages of 3, 7, 10, and 13 years. If stored in a polyethylene bottle, sodium fluoride is relatively stable. Sodium fluoride does not stain teeth, has an acceptable taste, and does not cause gingival inflammation. It is also supplied in a gel and a foam, which are applied using a disposable tray.

Stannous Fluoride

Stannous fluoride is an 8 or 10 percent aqueous solution applied once or twice annually. In some cases, where the caries index is high or where patients suffer from xerostomia (dry mouth) caused by prescription medications or systemic diseases or who are undergoing radiation or chemotherapy, stannous fluoride may be applied more often.

Stannous fluoride is highly unstable; a new solution must be dispensed or prepared for each application. It is unpleasant in taste and may stain demineralized areas of the teeth or porcelain or resin restorations. Stannous fluoride may cause sloughing of gingival tissues or gingivitis or aggravate certain periodontal conditions present during the time of application. Because of these adverse effects, stannous fluoride is rarely used today.

Acidulated Phosphate Fluoride (APF)

Acidulated phosphate fluoride is a 1.23 percent solution, gel, thixotropic gel, or foam with 0.1 M orthophosphoric acid. (A thixotropic gel becomes fluid when placed under stress, such as when it is forced interdentally or agitated in the container; it later returns to the original gel state.)

Acidulated phosphate fluoride is recommended for use twice annually. It is most optimally applied for 4 minutes; newer preparations only require 1-minute use, which is generally better tolerated by young children and patients with a gag reflex. Only the 4-minute application has the ADA seal of acceptance. Due to the orthophosphoric acid content, it may etch esthetic restorations in some patients' mouths. It is applied in single-use, disposable flexible trays (Figure 9-2).

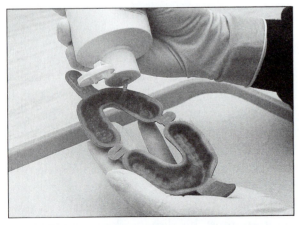

Figure 9-2 The dental assistant extrudes acidulated phosphate fluoride (APF) into a disposable tray.

Fluoride Varnish

Fluoride varnish (5 percent sodium fluoride) has been used as a desensitizing agent with a significant degree of success, primarily in Europe. Varnish is applied directly onto the surface of sensitive teeth, as directed by the dentist. (In some states it is legal for chairside assistants to apply desensitizing agents directly to tooth structures under the direct supervision of the dentist. Check with your state dental board to be sure.)

When properly applied, the solution remains on the tooth surface(s) for several hours, releasing fluoride into the immediate oral environment (especially the interproximal and cervical areas where it is most required).

For patients with continued dental sensitivity, reapplication may be indicated every six months. The sensitive tooth surface(s) are cleaned with pumice, then rinsed thoroughly with water. Excess water and saliva are removed using a three-way syringe. A thin layer of approximately 0.5 mm varnish is applied directly to the tooth or teeth using a disposable applicator brush. The varnish sets within a few seconds after contacting saliva. It leaves a fluoride-rich layer adjacent to the tooth surface. Prior to dismissal, the patient should be instructed to avoid brushing or eating for 2 hours following treatment as well as to abstain from using fluoride-containing mouth rinses for the remainder of the day.

■ SEALANTS

Pit and fissure sealants are another preventive dental material that may be recommended by the dentist, under certain clinical conditions, to help prevent caries from developing.

Applying Topical APF

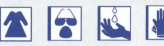

ARMAMENTARIUM

- Basic set-up
- Cotton rolls
- High-volume evacuation tip
- Saliva ejector
- Preformed commercial trays (either two single trays placed separately or two trays connected as one)
- Tray liners, if required by the manufacturer
- Fluoride gel
- Minute timer

PROCEDURE

Note that fluoride should be applied to clean, flossed teeth to be most effective.

1. Explain the procedure to the patient or to the accompanying parent if the patient is a young child.
2. Place the patient in an upright position to help prevent gagging.
3. Dispense the fluoride solution into the tray, filling to the amount recommended by the manufacturer.
4. Isolate the teeth with cotton rolls.
5. When treating both arches simultaneously, dry the maxillary arch first, then the mandibular.
6. Remove the cotton rolls and insert the tray(s) into the oral cavity (Figure 9-3). Use the thumb and index finger to squeeze the fluoride gel into the patient's interproximal areas.
7. Instruct the patient to close down gently so that all tooth surfaces are adequately covered by the fluoride. Insert the saliva ejector and set the timer to the

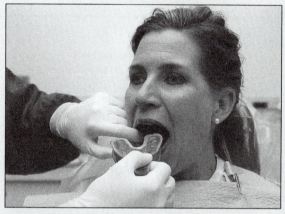

Figure 9-3 The dental assistant inserts the loaded fluoride tray into the patient's mouth.

appropriate number of minutes recommended by the manufacturer. (If the patient experiences a slight gag reflex, instruct him or her to tilt the head down slightly and to breathe through his or her nose.)

8. Use the saliva ejector or high-volume evacuation (HVE) tip inside the oral cavity to remove excess fluoride and/or saliva.
9. Remove the tray(s) after 4 minutes. Use the HVE or saliva ejector to suction out any remaining excess fluoride or saliva.
10. Instruct the patient not to swallow fluoride and not to rinse, eat, or drink for a minimum of 30 minutes. (This will allow the fluoride to be absorbed completely into the enamel.)

Use

Pit and fissure sealants are clinically indicated when there are deep pits and fissures in the occlusal surfaces of the posterior teeth that may be difficult to keep clean (Figure 9-4). They are occasionally recommended for deep pits in the lingual surfaces of upper lateral permanent incisors. While sealants are

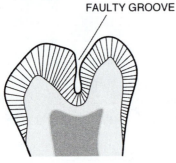

FAULTY GROOVE

Figure 9-4 Occlusal fissure showing deep pit, which is difficult for the patient to keep clean. Pit and fissure sealant is applied to the occlusal surfaces of posterior teeth.

most often applied to the teeth of children and adolescents, they are occasionally indicated in adults as well.

The sealant material bonds to the surface of the enamel and protects the tooth from accumulating bacteria that produce acids, which eventually start the caries process.

Pit and fissure sealants are most often indicated in the following clinical conditions:

- As a preventive measure to keep bacteria from entering deep crevices (pits and fissures) of teeth where Class I dental decay is most likely to develop
- On children's primary molars (there are no bicuspids in the deciduous dentition)
- On children with newly erupted permanent first molars

- Occasionally on pregnant women with elevated caries rates

Composition

There are three types of pit and fissure sealant: filled, unfilled, and fluoride-releasing filled. Sealants contain BIS-GMA resins; microparticles such as glass, quartz, and silica; and other fillers found in composite restorations that make them more resistant to occlusal abrasion. The polymer is an epoxy resin with an acrylic monomer, bisphenol A, and glycidyl methacrylate.

Sealants may be autopolymerized (self-cured) or photo cured (light cured).

Properties

The success of the sealant depends upon operator technique, the use of fresh materials, and the ability of the resin to complete adaptation to the tooth surface. Thus, the sealant should be of low viscosity for it to flow easily into the pits or fissures, allowing the material to contact the small surface irregularities of the tooth.

Mixing/Manipulation

Prior to placing a sealant, the tooth must be thoroughly cleaned, preferably using bicarbonate slurry solution with an air polisher. To ensure that the sealant has retentive properties,

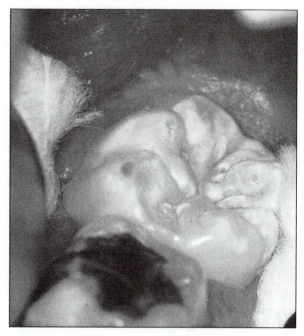

Figure 9-5 The acid-etched tooth takes on a chalky appearance.

the enamel surface must then be acid etched or conditioned, prior to placing the sealant. This is done using a concentrated solution of phosphoric acid (30–50 percent). Etching opens pores of the enamel surface to allow the sealant to flow into the surface irregularities to form resin tags. These resin tags create a mechanical interlocking of the resin to the enamel surface to increase bond strength to the tooth surface. Once etching is successfully completed, the tooth takes on a dull, white, chalky appearance (Figure 9-5).

PRACTICE MAKES PERFECT PROCEDURE ■ 9-2

Applying Pit and Fissure Sealant

ARMAMENTARIUM

- Basic set-up
- Cotton roll holders and cotton rolls or dental dam set-up
- Prophy brush, prophylaxis angle, and low-speed handpiece
- Flour of pumice and water or nonfluoridated prophy paste OR slurry bicarbonate solution and an air polisher
- HVE tip
- Saliva ejector
- Etchant/conditioner
- Sealant material: base material and catalyst (for self-cure) or base material (for light cure)
- Applicators (brush, small cotton pellets, or syringe for etch and sealant resin)
- Sealant dappen dish or disposable dappen dish supplied in sealant kit
- Light-curing unit (if required)
- Articulating paper and forceps
- Assorted burs and/or stones
- Dental floss
- Minute timer
- Protective eyewear for patient and dental personnel if a light-cured system is used
- Fluoride tray and fluoride for posttreatment (if indicated)

PROCEDURE

1. Explain the procedure to the patient or to the accompanying parent if he or she is a young child.
2. Polish the occlusal surface of each tooth to be sealed. Use flour of pumice or a nonfluoridated prophy paste on a bristle brush to thoroughly clean the occlusal surfaces. Or, an air polisher may be employed, using a bicarbonate slurry mixture. Rinse the tooth and thoroughly dry using oil-free compressed air.
3. Isolate the tooth to be sealed using either long and short cotton rolls or dental dam.
4. Redry the tooth to be sealed. Following the manufacturer's directions, apply the acid etchant/conditioner. Use an applicator to apply the etchant to the occlusal surface, into the pits and fissures and two-thirds up the cuspid incline. A gentle dabbing motion should be used to apply the etchant/conditioner for 60 seconds.
5. Rinse and dry the tooth; use the HVE tip to remove any residual water or acid etch material. Rinse for 20–30 seconds; redry the tooth for 20–30 seconds and reisolate with dry cotton rolls (if used).
6. The tooth should exhibit a dull, white, chalky appearance. If it does not, re-etch for another 15–30 seconds (Figure 9-5).
7. Following the manufacturer's instructions, apply the sealant material so that it flows into the pits and fissures and grooves of the tooth. Make sure that the material is not too thick. The material must flow properly into the tooth surfaces to allow these areas to be properly sealed. (The applicator tip or an explorer may be used to move the sealant into the pit and fissure areas and to prevent the formation of air bubbles.)
8. Allow the self-curing sealant to polymerize for the time recommended by the manufacturer. If using a light-cured sealant, hold the curing light 2 mm directly above the occlusal surface and expose the tooth for the appropriate time, generally 20–60 seconds.
9. Use an explorer to determine if the sealant is polymerized and smooth. It should be free of irregularities, voids, or air bubbles. If irregularities are found, the sealant process must be repeated to properly seal those areas. If the surface has been free of saliva, additional sealant may be added without re-etching the tooth. If saliva has contacted the tooth, however, the process must be repeated to prevent contamination.
10. After the sealant has set, rinse or wipe the occlusal surface using a cotton roll or pellet moistened with water.
11. Remove cotton rolls and holder or dental dam. Check the tooth contacts with floss, looking for excess sealant material.
12. Dry the sealed tooth and use articulating paper to check for high spots on the sealant. If marks are dark from the articulating paper, the operator may use a bur or stone to reduce them. Often, these high areas wear down within a few days as a result of the patient's chewing patterns. If filled sealant material is used, high spots should be removed.
13. Instruct the patient not to eat or chew for at least 30 minutes on the side(s) where the sealant material was applied. Also inform the patient that chewing ice, eating foods with acid such as lemons, and drinking soft drinks may break the bond over a period of time. Inform the patient that with proper care and diet, sealants last about two years.

Special Considerations

- Take care not to allow saliva or other moisture to contaminate the working field.
- Do not allow etching material to contact clothing, eyes, skin, or the oral mucosa.
- Always wear PPE when working at chairside.
- Maintain and work in a clean, dry, aseptic field.
- Clean and disinfect the work area at the conclusion of the procedure, after dismissing the patient.
- Always follow OSHA regulations and CDC recommendations to help prevent the spread of bloodborne diseases and to protect dental personnel.

▪ TOOTH BLEACHING

Tooth bleaching (whitening) is a relatively new cosmetic dental procedure. Dental bleaching is broken down into three categories: nonvital (in-office), active vital (in-office), and passive vital (performed by the patient at home under the supervision of the dentist). Some patients undergo two types of dental bleaching (active and passive) simultaneously.

Use

Nonvital tooth bleaching is performed in the office by the dentist on endodontically treated teeth, that is, those having undergone root canal therapy. Endodontically treated teeth often become discolored following treatment as a result of blood, restorative materials used to fill the canal, or accumulation of pulpal debris. This procedure is often referred to as "walking bleach technique."

Vital tooth bleaching is performed in the office using bleaching liquids or gels, most often accelerated using a curing light or other heating device. This is referred to as "power bleaching."

Passive vital bleaching requires the patient to wear custom-fabricated trays or stents, most often during sleep, that hold a bleaching solution or gel. The result depends upon how long or how often the patient wears the stent filled with bleaching material.

Composition

Tooth bleaching is accomplished using a variety of bleach with other additives. Nonvital tooth bleaching, or walking bleach technique, is performed using a thick paste of hydrogen peroxide, sodium perborate, or a combination of the two placed into the coronal portion of the nonvital tooth. The bleach mixture is then temporarily sealed in place and the patient is reappointed to evaluate the degree of tooth whiteness in relation to the adjacent teeth. In some cases, the dentist will elect to apply external heat to the nonvital tooth during bleaching to accelerate the whitening process.

During vital in-office bleaching (power bleaching), the bleaching liquid or gel is often applied in combination with a heat lamp or curing light. The patient's teeth are isolated with dental dam to prevent gingival irritation from the bleaching chemicals and then polished with prophy paste or pumice. The bleaching material, depending upon the manufacturer, is sometimes applied sometimes several times during a 1-hour procedure and then the heat or light source is administered.

In between each addition of bleaching material, the teeth are washed and dried and evaluated by the dentist to determine the desired result. Once the desired result has been achieved and agreed upon by the patient, the dental dam is removed and the newly bleached teeth are polished using a fluoride prophy paste. The patient may be rescheduled several weeks later for evaluation; he or she should be advised that the teeth may be somewhat sensitive following the appointment and that extremely hot or cold beverages should be avoided temporarily until the sensitivity diminishes. Custom fluoride trays are sometimes given to the patient for home application to help reduce tooth sensitivity.

Passive vital bleaching is done by the patient at home under the supervision of the dentist. The patient applies a bleaching solution, most often carbamide peroxide or diluted hydrogen peroxide, in a custom-fitted tray or stent. Some patients may begin their passive bleaching process by first scheduling one start-up appointment, sometimes referred to as "assisted bleaching," and then completing the self-administered applications.

In addition to the passive vital bleaching done under the supervision of the dentist, many other home bleaching products have been introduced to customers. Patients may have questions regarding these products when they visit the dentist. Home bleaching systems come in several different forms. One popular form includes strips which are peeled and applied to the teeth. Strips have a low percentage of hydrogen peroxide. Another bleaching system is whitening toothpaste. These toothpastes also have a low percentage of hydrogen peroxide and must be used for a certain length of time before noticeable results are evident. Home bleaching is also available with moldable trays and whitening gel syringes which contain hydrogen peroxide. Regardless of the bleaching system used, patients may experience some sensitivity (usually temporary) to their teeth.

PRACTICE MAKES PERFECT PROCEDURE ▪ 9-3

In-Office Nonvital Tooth Bleaching

ARMAMENTARIUM
- Basic set-up
- Cotton rolls, 2 × 2 gauze sponges, cotton pellets
- HVE tip, air-water three-way syringe, saliva ejector
- Dental dam set-up
- Protective gel or petroleum jelly
- Waxed dental floss
- High-speed handpiece with assorted burs
- Rubber polishing cup, prophy paste, prophylaxis angle, and low-speed handpiece
- Cement-base materials
- Bleaching kit materials
- Light-curing unit or heat lamp
- Temporary cement
- Finishing burs
- Timer

PROCEDURE
1. Dental dam is placed on the appropriate teeth. Protective gel is applied underneath the dam and then again along the inverted edges of the dam to create an effective seal.
2. The dentist removes the access restoration and debris inside.
3. The dentist cleans the chamber of the open tooth using a prophy brush or cotton pellet.
4. If the in-office (only) technique is used, the dentist fills the pulp chamber through lingual or occlusal access of the tooth with bleaching for 30 minutes, replacing the gel every 10 minutes, taking care not to let the bleaching gel penetrate the root, as this makes it brittle and more likely to fracture. The dentist may use the heat lamp or curing light to facilitate bleaching. A cotton pellet and temporary cement or temporary crown are placed on the tooth and the patient is reappointed for reevaluation in three to seven days.
5. If the walking bleach technique is used, the dentist places a thick mixture of bleaching agent in the crown and covers it with temporary cement. The patient is reappointed in two to five days for reevaluation and to remove the cotton pellet.
6. The final restoration is polished with the high-speed handpiece and finishing burs.

Properties

Dental bleaching materials may cause tooth sensitivity to the affected areas as well as gingival irritation or sloughing of tissue. Patients should avoid overbleaching, as this may also desiccate (dry out) tooth enamel.

PRACTICE MAKES PERFECT PROCEDURE ▪ 9-4

In-Office Vital (Active) Tooth Bleaching

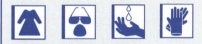

ARMAMENTARIUM

- Basic set-up
- Protective gel or petroleum jelly
- Dental dam set-up
- Waxed floss
- Low-speed handpiece, prophy brush, or cup and composite resin or fluoride prophy paste
- Bleaching kit
- Heat lamp or curing light
- Minute timer

PROCEDURE

1. Apply protective gel or petroleum jelly to surrounding areas of teeth to receive bleach.
2. Apply dental dam, placing a ligature of waxed floss around each tooth.
3. Gently polish each tooth to remove plaque and debris that could interfere with the bleaching procedure using prophy paste or flour of pumice. A shade should be taken at this point, prior to bleaching.
4. Follow the manufacturer's instructions for use of materials and placement of bleaching materials. Note that some bleaching materials require a heat lamp or light source and are used for 30 minutes. No-heat materials are applied every 10 minutes using new solution using fresh materials mixed each time for three or four applications. The teeth must be rinsed, evacuated, and dried between each application.
5. When satisfactory whitening has been achieved, thoroughly rinse the area, cut the ligatures, and remove interseptal dental dam.
6. Rinse again, removing any remaining gel with floss and dampened gauze.
7. Instruct the patient to avoid substances that may cause staining of enamel, also that the teeth may be somewhat sensitive. Reschedule for several more active bleaching appointments, usually several weeks apart.

Special Considerations

- Do not allow bleaching material to contact clothing, oral mucosa, skin, or eyes.
- Take extra care not to let the bleaching light burn the patient's skin or oral mucosa.
- Instruct the patient about dental sensitivity associated with tooth bleaching.
- Always wear PPE when working at chairside.
- Maintain and work in a clean, dry, aseptic field.
- Clean and disinfect the work area at the conclusion of the procedure, after dismissing the patient.
- Always follow OSHA regulations and CDC recommendations to help prevent the spread of bloodborne diseases and to protect dental personnel.

Mixing/Manipulation

Tooth bleaching materials are supplied premixed and ready to use. Where trays or stents are required for passive vital bleaching at home, the patient must have alginate impressions made, from which stone models are poured. A custom tray is then fashioned over the tooth model(s), most often using a vacuum-forming device (see Chapter 8: Dental Resins for additional information on how to make a vacuum-formed tray).

PRACTICE MAKES PERFECT PROCEDURE ▪ 9-5

Passive (Home) Tooth Bleaching

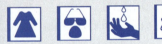

ARMAMENTARIUM
- Basic set-up
- Alginate set-up
- Mixing bowl and spatula
- Alginate impression trays
- Vacuum-formed tray material, spacer material, and vacuum-forming machine
- Home bleaching kit with home care instructions
- Shade guide for before and after color comparison

PROCEDURE
1. Take alginate impressions of the arches to be bleached. (Note that some practices recommend bleaching only the maxillary teeth.) Some practices also take "before" and "after" photographs for whitening comparison.
2. Dismiss and reappoint the patient.

Between Appointments
3. Pour the impressions in model stone and trim.
4. Fashion a custom tray or stent for each arch to be bleached. (Note that the dental assistant should check the manufacturer's directions to determine if spacer material should be placed to allow room for the beaching solution or gel.)
5. Examine the edges of the trays for roughness and smooth accordingly.

Second Appointment
6. Check the tray(s) for patient comfort and fit.
7. Give home care instructions and bleaching solution/gel and ask the patient to practice inserting the tray(s).
8. Dismiss the patient and reappoint for follow-up and color evaluation.

■ PERIODONTAL SURGICAL DRESSING MATERIALS

In addition to being familiar with preventive dental materials, the dental assistant must be familiar with **periodontal surgical dressings**.

Use

A periodontal dressing is placed over the site of the surgical wound to act as a bandage during the healing process. At the completion of the periodontal surgical procedure and after hemorrhaging has been controlled, the periodontal dressing is placed. The surgical site must be as dry as possible for the dressing to adhere properly.

In some states the dental assistant may apply and remove periodontal dressings; in others, only the licensed dentist (or hygienist) may perform this procedure.

Composition

There are three types of periodontal dressings: zinc oxide–eugenol, noneugenol, and light cured. Some manufacturers supply periodontal dressing already mixed; others supply it in tubes of base and accelerator, which require mixing.

In some practices where large quantities of periodontal surgical dressing are used, the dental assistant may mix larger quantities of the periodontal surgical dressing ahead of time and store it in the refrigerator. A sufficient quantity should be taken out of the refrigerator prior to the surgical patient's appointment.

Properties

As the material is mixed, it becomes sticky or tacky. It is placed in a paper cup filled with cool water to reach a malleable consistency, without tackiness.

Mixing/Manipulation

The dental assistant extrudes equal lengths of base and accelerator onto the large paper mixing pad supplied by the manufacturer. The two items should be extruded next to each other on the pad but not touching until the dentist or periodontist gives instructions to begin mixing. The dental assistant uses a wooden tongue depressor to gather up the material and mix it together until homogenous.

The material is then gathered up onto the tongue depressor and placed into a cup of cold water.

After the mixture reaches a tacky consistency, it is rolled onto the mixing pad and the material shaped into thin tubes by rolling it between the fingers.

The rope of periodontal surgical dressing is then applied to the facial surface of the gingiva, equivalent to the length of the incision of the wound, beginning at the distal of the most posterior tooth and working forward. When correctly applied, the periodontal dressing should cover the incision and the gingival one-third of the tooth, including part of gingiva toward the apical side, but without interfering with muscle attachments. It should extend mesially and distally one tooth beyond the surgical incision. The dressing is then mechanically locked and festooned (shaped) in the interproximal area with a plastic placement instrument and/or moist cotton-tipped applicator. The total width of the dressing should be less than 6 mm.

A second rope of periodontal surgical dressing is then added to the lingual side, beginning at the distal and working forward. A plastic placement instrument is used to lock the material interproximally around the gingival one-third of each tooth to provide somewhat of an esthetic appearance.

PRACTICE MAKES PERFECT PROCEDURE ■ 9-6

Placing Noneugenol Periodontal Dressing

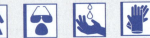

ARMAMENTARIUM
- Basic set-up
- Plastic placement instrument
- 2 × 2 gauze sponges
- Tongue depressors for mixing the periodontal surgical dressing
- Large paper mixing pad
- Periodontal dressing base and accelerator
- Cotton-tipped applicators
- Water-based lubricant, such as KY jelly
- Saline solution
- Cup filled with cold water
- Gelfoam

PROCEDURE
1. Dispense sufficient lengths of base and accelerator onto the large paper mixing pad, according to the manufacturer's instructions.
2. At the direction of the dentist or periodontist, use a tongue depressor to incorporate the materials together until a homogenous mixture is achieved.
3. Gather up and place the mixed material on the tip of the tongue depressor and place it into a cup of cold water (Figure 9-6).

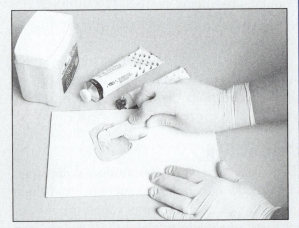

Figure 9-6 The dental assistant uses a tongue depressor and large paper pad to incorporate the periodontal surgical dressing.

4. Apply lubricant to coat the patient's lips and the operator's (or dental assistant's) gloves.

5. Use 2 × 2 gauze sponges to check the surgical site to ensure that bleeding has stopped and blot to ensure that excess saliva has been removed. If sutures have been placed, locate the knots and cover them with Gelfoam to avoid embedding them in the dressing.

6. When the periodontal surgical dressing mixture has lost its tacky consistency, remove it and roll it out onto the mixing pad.

7. Take the material in gloved hands and roll it into thin ropes (Figure 9-7).

8. Begin adapting the rope of material to the facial side, starting at the posterior and working forward (Figure 9-8). Use a plastic placement instrument and/or moist cotton-tipped applicator to mechanically bond the dressing interproximally (Figure 9-9).

9. Repeat on the lingual surface, covering approximately the gingival one-third of each tooth.

10. The dentist or periodontist checks the patient's occlusion.

11. Clean the patient's face; dismiss and reappoint him or her. Give the patient a postoperative appointment and necessary postoperative instructions and prescriptions.

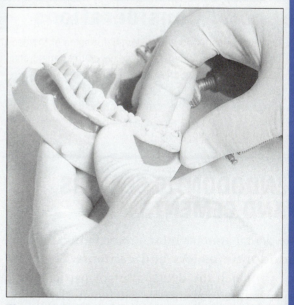

Figure 9-8 Placement of periodontal surgical dressing demonstrated on a typodont.

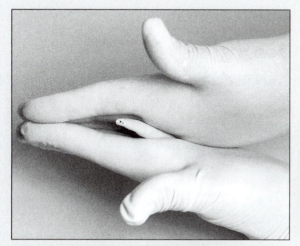

Figure 9-7 The dental assistant rolls the periodontal surgical dressing into "ropes" for application to the facial and lingual sides of the teeth involved.

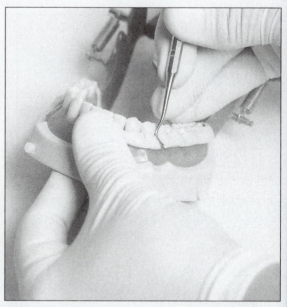

Figure 9-9 Demonstration using a plastic instrument to "tuck" the periodontal surgical dressing interproximally for mechanical retention.

■ ENDODONTIC SEALERS AND CEMENTS

The dental assistant must also be familiar with **endodontic sealers and cements**. The extent to which the dental assistant participates in procedures that involve these materials (see "Use" below) will depend partially on the dental assistant's state of employment.

Use

Root canal sealing materials are used by the dentist to prevent microleakage inside the canal(s) of a tooth being endodontically treated.

Composition

Root canal sealers are supplied in a variety of compositions, including zinc oxide–eugenol, calcium hydroxide, and glass ionomer. Their format may include powders and liquids, pastes, or capsules (Figure 9-10).

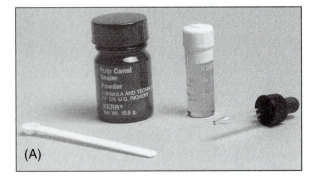

(A)

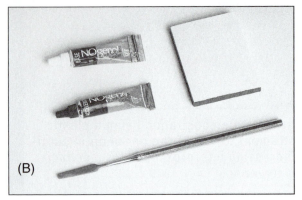

(B)

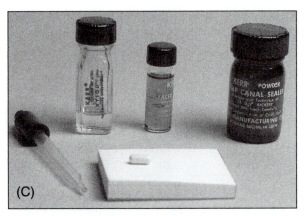

(C)

Figure 9-10 Root canal sealers: (A) powder and liquid; (B) two-paste system; (C) capsules.

■ CRITICAL THINKING QUESTIONS

1. Why should the dental assistant instruct the patient not to swallow fluoride and not to rinse, eat, or drink for a minimum of 30 minutes following completion of treatment?
2. What is the significance of a dull, white, chalky appearance of the tooth enamel as part of the pit and fissure sealant application procedure?
3. Why is spacer material necessary when fashioning a custom vacuum-formed bleaching tray (stent)?
4. Why is the periodontal surgical dressing shaped into thin ropes?

PRACTICE MAKES PERFECT
STUDENT ASSESSMENT 9-1

Applying Topical APF

Student's Name: _____

Date: _____   Instructor: _____

Note: The blank space is provided for the instructor to check off the student's progress. The student may practice the procedure as many times as necessary before being evaluated. Some portions of the exercise may be performed on a typodont, stone tooth model, or extracted tooth or simulated in a clinical operatory. The student has successfully completed the following:

_____ Worn necessary PPE

_____ Assembled necessary armamentarium

_____ Maintained a clear, dry, aseptic working field

_____ Explained the procedure to the patient or to the accompanying parent if he or she was a young child

_____ Placed the patient in an upright position

_____ Dispensed the fluoride solution into the tray, filling to the amount recommended by the manufacturer

_____ Isolated the teeth with cotton rolls

_____ Dried the maxillary arch first

_____ Removed the cotton rolls and inserted the tray(s) into the oral cavity

_____ Used the thumb and index finger to squeeze the fluoride gel into the patient's interproximal areas

_____ Instructed the patient to close down gently so that all tooth surfaces were adequately covered by the fluoride

_____ Inserted the saliva ejector and set the timer to the appropriate number of minutes (4) recommended by the manufacturer

_____ Used the saliva ejector or HVE tip inside the oral cavity to remove excess fluoride and/or saliva

_____ Removed the tray(s) after the appropriate time had elapsed (4 minutes)

_____ Used the HVE or saliva ejector to suction out any remaining excess fluoride or saliva

_____ Instructed the patient not to swallow fluoride and not to rinse, eat, or drink for a minimum of 30 minutes

_____ Cleaned and disinfected the work area at the conclusion of the procedure, after dismissing the patient

_____ Followed OSHA regulations and CDC recommendations to help prevent the spread of bloodborne diseases and to protect dental personnel

Comments

_____

_____

_____

_____

_____

Applying Pit and Fissure Sealant

Student's Name: _____

Date: _____   Instructor: _____

Note: The blank space is provided for the instructor to check off the student's progress. The student may practice the procedure as many times as necessary before being evaluated. Some portions of the exercise may be performed on a typodont, stone tooth model, or extracted tooth or simulated in a clinical operatory. The student has successfully completed the following:

_____ Worn necessary PPE

_____ Assembled necessary armamentarium

_____ Maintained a clear, dry, aseptic working field

_____ Explained the procedure to the patient or to the accompanying parent if he or she was a young child

_____ Cleansed the occlusal surface of each tooth to be sealed; used flour of pumice or a nonfluoridated prophy paste with bristle brush or bicarbonate slurry and air polisher to thoroughly clean the occlusal surfaces; rinsed the teeth and thoroughly dried, using oil-free compressed air

_____ Isolated the teeth to be sealed using either long and short cotton rolls or dental dam

_____ Redried the teeth to be sealed

_____ Following the manufacturer's directions, applied the acid etchant/conditioner; used an applicator to apply the etchant to the occlusal surface, into the pits and fissures and two-thirds up the cuspid incline using a gentle dabbing motion for 60 seconds

_____ Rinsed the teeth for 20–30 seconds; used the HVE tip to remove any residual water or acid

_____ Redried the teeth for 20–30 seconds and reisolated them with dry cotton rolls (if used)

_____ If the teeth did not exhibit a dull, white, chalky appearance, re-etched them for another 15–30 seconds

_____ Following the manufacturer's instructions, applied the sealant material so it flowed into the pits and fissures and reached the desired thickness (The applicator tip or an explorer may have been used to move the sealant into the pit and fissure areas and to prevent the formation of air bubbles.)

_____ Allowed the self-curing sealant to polymerize for the time recommended by the manufacturer; if using a light-cured sealant, held the curing light 2 mm directly above the occlusal surface and exposed the tooth for the appropriate time (20–60 seconds)

_____ Used an explorer to determine that the sealant was polymerized and smooth; if irregularities were found, repeated the sealant process to properly seal those areas

_____ After the sealant set, rinsed or wiped the surface using a moist cotton roll or pellet

_____ Removed cotton rolls and holder or dental dam; checked the tooth contacts with floss, looking for excess sealant material

_____ Dried the sealed teeth and used articulating paper to check for high spots on the sealant; if necessary, reduced them

_____ Administered topical fluoride treatment (if indicated)

_____ Instructed the patient not to eat or chew on the side(s) where the sealant material was applied

_____ Cleaned and disinfected the work area at the conclusion of the procedure, after dismissing the patient

_____ Followed OSHA regulations and CDC recommendations to help prevent the spread of bloodborne diseases and to protect dental personnel

Comments

_____

_____

_____

_____

_____

In-Office Nonvital Tooth Bleaching

Student's Name: _____

Date: _____   Instructor: _____

Note: The blank space is provided for the instructor to check off the student's progress. The student may practice the procedure as many times as necessary before being evaluated. Some portions of the exercise may be performed on a typodont, stone tooth model, or extracted tooth or simulated in a clinical operatory. The student has successfully completed the following:

_____ Worn necessary PPE

_____ Assembled necessary armamentarium

_____ Maintained a clear, dry, aseptic working field

_____ Placed dental dam on the appropriate teeth

_____ Applied protective gel underneath the dam and along the inverted edges of the dam to create an effective seal

_____ The dentist removed the access restoration and debris inside

_____ Taken and recorded shade using shade guide

_____ The dentist cleaned the chamber of the open tooth using a prophy brush or cotton pellet

_____ If the in-office (only) technique was used, the dentist filled the pulp chamber through lingual or occlusal access of the tooth with bleaching for 30 minutes, replacing the gel every 10 minutes, taking care not to let the bleaching gel penetrate the root; a cotton pellet and temporary cement were placed in the tooth and the patient was reappointed for reevaluation

_____ If the walking bleach technique was used, the dentist placed a thick mixture of bleaching agent in the pulp chamber of the crown and covered it with temporary cement; the patient was reappointed in two to five days for reevaluation and for removal of the cotton pellet

_____ Polished the final restoration with the high-speed handpiece and finishing burs

_____ Cleaned and disinfected the work area at the conclusion of the procedure, after dismissing the patient

_____ Followed OSHA regulations and CDC recommendations to help prevent the spread of bloodborne diseases and to protect dental personnel

Comments

_____

_____

_____

_____

_____

In-Office Vital (Active) Tooth Bleaching

Student's Name: _____

Date: _____   Instructor: _____

Note: The blank space is provided for the instructor to check off the student's progress. The student may practice the procedure as many times as necessary before being evaluated. Some portions of the exercise may be performed on a typodont, stone tooth model, or extracted tooth or simulated in a clinical operatory. The student has successfully completed the following:

_____ Worn necessary PPE

_____ Assembled necessary armamentarium

_____ Maintained a clear, dry, aseptic working field

_____ Applied dental dam on the appropriate teeth

_____ Applied protective gel or petroleum jelly to surrounding areas of teeth to receive bleach

_____ Gently polished each tooth to remove plaque and debris that could interfere with the bleaching procedure using prophy paste or flour of pumice

_____ Took and recorded tooth shade using shade guide

_____ Followed the manufacturer's instructions for use and placement of bleaching materials

_____ When satisfactory whitening was achieved, thoroughly rinsed the area, cut the ligatures, and removed interseptal dental dam segments

_____ Rinsed the teeth again, removing any remaining gel with floss and dampened gauze

_____ Instructed the patient to avoid substances that might cause staining of enamel, also that the teeth may be somewhat sensitive

_____ Rescheduled the patient for next bleaching appointment

_____ Cleaned and disinfected the work area at the conclusion of the procedure, after dismissing the patient

_____ Followed OSHA regulations and CDC recommendations to help prevent the spread of bloodborne diseases and to protect dental personnel

Comments

_____

_____

_____

_____

_____

Passive (Home) Tooth Bleaching

Student's Name: _____

Date: _____   Instructor: _____

Note: The blank space is provided for the instructor to check off the student's progress. The student may practice the procedure as many times as necessary before being evaluated. Some portions of the exercise may be performed on a typodont, stone tooth model, or extracted tooth or simulated in a clinical operatory. The student has successfully completed the following:

_____ Worn necessary PPE
_____ Assembled necessary armamentarium
_____ Maintained a clear, dry, aseptic working field
_____ Took alginate impressions of the arch(es) to receive bleach

Between Appointments

_____ Poured and trimmed the stone models
_____ Fashioned a custom tray or stent for each arch to be bleached (The dental assistant placed spacer material to allow room for the beaching solution or gel, if required.)
_____ Examined the edges of the tray(s) for roughness and smoothed them accordingly

Second Appointment

_____ Checked the tray(s) for patient comfort and fit
_____ Gave the patient home care instructions and bleaching solution or gel and asked to practice inserting the tray(s)
_____ Dismissed the patient and reappointed for a follow-up appointment and color evaluation
_____ Cleaned and disinfected the work area at the conclusion of the procedure, after dismissing the patient.
_____ Followed OSHA regulations and CDC recommendations to help prevent the spread of bloodborne diseases and to protect dental personnel

Comments

_____

_____

_____

_____

_____

PRACTICE MAKES PERFECT
STUDENT ASSESSMENT 9-6

Placing Noneugenol Periodontal Dressing

Student's Name: _____

Date: _____ Instructor: _____

Note: The blank space is provided for the instructor to check off the student's progress. The student may practice the procedure as many times as necessary before being evaluated. Some portions of the exercise may be performed on a typodont, stone tooth model, or extracted tooth or simulated in a clinical operatory. The student has successfully completed the following:

_____ Worn necessary PPE

_____ Assembled necessary armamentarium

_____ Maintained a clear, dry, aseptic working field

_____ Dispensed sufficient lengths of base and accelerator onto the large paper mixing pad, according to the manufacturer's instructions

_____ At the direction of the dentist or periodontist, used a tongue depressor to incorporate the materials together until a homogenous mixture was achieved

_____ Gathered up and placed the mixed material on the tip of the tongue depressor and placed it into a cup of cold water

_____ Applied lubricant to coat the patient's lips and the operator's (or dental assistant's) gloves

_____ Used 2 × 2 gauze sponges to check the surgical site to ensure that bleeding had stopped and blotted to ensure that excess saliva had been removed; if sutures had been placed, located the knots and covered them with Gelfoam to avoid embedding them in the dressing

_____ When the periodontal surgical dressing mixture had lost its tacky consistency, removed it and rolled it out onto the mixing pad

_____ Took the material in gloved hands and rolled it into thin ropes

_____ Adapted the rope of material to the facial side, starting at the posterior and working forward

_____ Used a plastic placement instrument and/or moist cotton-tipped applicator to mechanically bond and festooned the dressing interproximally

_____ Repeated on the lingual surface, covering approximately the gingival one-third of each tooth

_____ The dentist or periodontist checked the patient's occlusion

_____ Cleaned the patient's face and dismissed and reappointed him or her; gave the patient a postoperative appointment and necessary postoperative instructions and prescriptions

_____ Cleaned and disinfected the work area at the conclusion of the procedure, after dismissing the patient

_____ Followed OSHA regulations and CDC recommendations to help prevent the spread of bloodborne diseases and to protect dental personnel

Comments

_____

_____

_____

_____

_____

CHAPTER 9: POSTTEST

Instructions: For each of the following, select the answer that most accurately completes the question or statement.

1. The optimal level of fluoride is _____ (ppm), delivered in most community/public water systems.
   A. 1 part per million
   B. 5 parts per million
   C. 10 parts per million
   D. 100 parts per million

2. Acidulated phosphate fluoride (APF) is a _____ solution, gel, or thixotropic form with 0.1 M orthophosphoric acid.
   A. 2%
   B. 8%
   C. 1.23%
   D. 15.23%

3. The recommended application time for stannous and acidulated phosphate fluorides is
   A. at ages 3, 7, 10, and 13 years
   B. once annually
   C. once every three months
   D. once every six months

4. All of the following are true with regard to stannous fluoride *except* it
   A. is highly unstable
   B. is highly stable
   C. has an unpleasant taste
   D. may stain demineralized areas of the teeth or tooth-colored permanent restorations
   E. may aggravate certain periodontal conditions

5. All of the following are true regarding acidulated phosphate fluoride (APF) *except* it
   A. is a 1.23% solution, gel, or thixotropic form with 0.1 M orthophosphoric acid
   B. is generally recommended for application every six months
   C. is recommended for application at ages 3, 7, 10, and 13 years
   D. may be applied for either 1 or 4 minutes, depending upon the manufacturer's instructions
   E. is applied in single-use, disposable, flexible trays

6. All of the following are types of pit and fissure sealant *except*
   A. filled
   B. unfilled
   C. time released
   D. fluoride-releasing filled

7. Sealants may be
   A. autopolymerized (self cured)
   B. photocured (light cured)
   C. photosynthesized cured
   D. A and B only
   E. A, B, and C

8. Pit and fissure sealant material should be of _____ viscosity for it to flow easily into the pits or fissures, allowing the material to contact the small surface irregularities of the tooth.
   A. low
   B. medium
   C. high
   D. ultrahigh

9. The enamel surface must be acid etched prior to placing a sealant so as to
   A. provide additional fluoride to the tooth or teeth
   B. ensure that the sealant has retentive properties
   C. ensure that the photo-cure light will function properly
   D. prevent air bubbles from forming in the sealant material

10. Acid etching opens pores of the enamel surface to allow the sealant to flow into the surface irregularities forming resin tags, which create a mechanical interlocking of the resin to the enamel surface. This results in
    A. increased bond strength to the tooth's surface
    B. a dull, white, chalky appearance
    C. a deep, violet color
    D. A and B only
    E. B and C only
    F. A, B, and C

11. Acid etching is accomplished using a _____ acid solution.
    A. 10–20% phosphoric
    B. 30–50% phosphoric
    C. 10–20% boric
    D. 30–50% boric

12. How may the teeth to receive pit and fissure sealant material be isolated prior to beginning the procedure?
    A. garmer cotton roll holders with long and short cotton rolls
    B. dental dam
    C. waxed dental floss
    D. either A or B only
    E. A, B, or C

13. Nonvital tooth bleaching is performed
    A. in the office on teeth prior to receiving endodontic treatment
    B. at home by the patient, under the supervision of the dentist
    C. in the office by the dentist on teeth following completion of endodontic treatment
    D. on deciduous teeth only

14. The technique of vital tooth bleaching performed in the office using bleaching liquids or gels and accelerated using a curing light or other heating device is often referred to as
    A. passive bleaching
    B. selective bleaching
    C. power bleaching
    D. emphatic bleaching

15. _____ bleaching requires the patient to wear custom-fabricated trays or stents, most often during sleep, that hold a bleaching solution or gel. The result depends upon how long or how often the patient wears the stent filled with bleaching material.
    A. Passive
    B. Active
    C. Nonvital
    D. Power

16.. The patient undergoing tooth bleaching should be advised of all of the following *except*
    A. An evaluation appointment will be scheduled several weeks later.
    B. The teeth may be somewhat sensitive.
    C. Hot and cold foods and beverages should be avoided temporarily.
    D. Foods and beverages that tend to stain enamel should be avoided.
    E. No further appointments are necessary.

17. Which of the following statements are true with regard to passive vital tooth bleaching?
    A. Passive vital bleaching is done by the patient at home under the supervision of the dentist.
    B. The patient applies a bleaching solution, most often carbamide peroxide or diluted hydrogen peroxide, in a custom-fitted tray or stent.
    C. Some patients may begin their passive bleaching process by first scheduling one start-up appointment, sometimes referred to as "assisted bleaching."
    D. A and B only
    E. B and C only
    F. All of the above

18. What is the purpose of a heat lamp or curing light in tooth whitening?
    A. to avoid having the patient undergo endodontic therapy
    B. to facilitate the bleaching process
    C. to retard the bleaching process
    D. to activate the acid-etch gel

19. If the walking bleach technique is used, the dentist places a thick mixture of bleaching agent in the crown and covers it with temporary cement. The patient is reappointed in two to five days for reevaluation and to remove the cotton pellet.
    A. True
    B. False

20. What is the purpose of placing a periodontal dressing?
    A. It helps facilitate the acid-etch process.
    B. It prevents teeth from becoming stained.
    C. It seals root canals.
    D. It is placed over the site of the surgical wound to act as a bandage during the healing process.

MISCELLANEOUS DENTAL MATERIALS AND HAZARDOUS SUBSTANCES

LEARNING OBJECTIVES

Upon completion of this chapter the student should be able to:

1. Describe and relate miscellaneous occupational materials and substances used by the dental assistant.

2. Relate methods and procedures to work with these materials for his or her safety, the safety of patients, and the safety of all dental team members.

3. Describe safety practices associated with the use of gases in the dental office.

4. Describe the dental assistant's role in the proper use of darkroom chemistry materials and related waste management.

5. Describe the importance of a hazard communication program in the dental office and the necessary components, including physical and chemical hazards, Material Safety Data Sheets (MSDSs), required staff training and documentation, and methods to reduce hazards in the dental office.

KEY TERMS

biohazard warning labels
chlorine dioxide
   compounds
developer
ethylene oxide
fixer
glutaraldehydes
hazard communication
   program
hazardous materials log
iodophors
isopropyl alcohol
nitrous oxide
phenolics
radiographs (x-rays)
sodium hypochlorite

■ INTRODUCTION

The dental assistant encounters a number of potentially hazardous miscellaneous occupational materials and substances in the dental office. It is important that the dental assistant, whether working in the front office handling business management duties or working in the clinical areas, be familiar with these substances, their potential hazards, special handling, storage, labeling, documentation procedures, and precautions.

Dental assistants interested in additional information on this subject may wish to refer to Chapter 14: Occupational Environmental Hazards in *Safety Standards and Infection Control for Dental Assistants* (by E. Dietz, 2002, Clifton Park, NY: Thomson Delmar Learning).

■ CHEMICAL DISINFECTANTS AND STERILANTS

A number of chemical disinfectants are available (Box 10-1) to the dental assistant for use on environmental surfaces and equipment that cannot be sterilized. Disinfectants may be harmful if inhaled excessively or used in areas with inadequate ventilation. The dental assistant should always use disinfecting chemicals with great caution, taking care not to spill, splash, or inhale them. Skin and clothing contact with disinfectants should also be avoided because this may cause stinging, burning of

---

DID YOU KNOW?

When working with chemical sterilants, the dental assistant must be careful to avoid directly touching the solutions, unnecessarily splashing the solutions, or breathing in their vapors to minimize health risks.

The dental assistant must always take special care when handling chemical sterilants and disinfectants because of their toxicity:

- Always wear appropriate PPE.
- Always follow the manufacturer's instructions for storing, diluting, handling, and disposal.
- Never allow solutions to touch intact skin, to contact the eyes, or to be inhaled.
- Follow instructions for proper shelf life and use life (term of usage) and dispose of all solutions according to local statutes and government requirements.
- Keep necessary clean-up and spill-kit materials handy in the event of an accidental spill or splashing of solutions.

Box 10-1 Guidelines for Mixing, Handling, and Discarding Chemical Sterilants and Disinfectants

the eyes, skin, or lungs, or permanent discoloration of clothing.

Chlorine Dioxide Compounds

Chlorine dioxide compounds are EPA-registered, high-level chemical disinfectants (and sterilants) that can be used only on instruments, environmental surfaces, and equipment not susceptible to corrosion. Items that are corrosive are those made of or containing high amounts of stainless steel, carbide steel, copper, or brass. Because of this corrosive property, chlorine dioxide disinfectants should be stored only in plastic or glass containers.

As with using any disinfectant, the dental assistant should always follow the manufacturer's instructions for handling and storage as well as disposal.

Chlorine dioxide compounds may also be used for processing instruments; when used as an instrument sterilant, from 6 to 10 hours is required, which may not be practical.

Glutaraldehydes

Glutaraldehydes are EPA–registered, high-level disinfectants (and sterilants) that may also have a corrosive effect upon certain metals. Thus, the dental assistant must exercise caution when using them.

Glutaraldehydes may also be used for processing instruments; disinfection time with glutaraldehydes takes from 10 to 90 minutes; sterilization takes 6–10 hours, which may not be practical. (Glutaraldehyde does not have a residual effect.)

The dental assistant must note that if additional instruments or related items are added to the glutaraldehyde solution, the "start" time must begin again. (Glutaraldehydes retain efficacy for 28 days from the time of mixing, even if not used.)

As when handling, mixing, storing, and disposing of all chemicals, the dental assistant must follow the manufacturer's instructions.

Also used as an ingredient in x-ray developers, glutaraldehyde has been associated with skin, eye, and respiratory irritation as well as allergic contact dermatitis, headaches, nausea, nosebleed, mucous membrane irritation, and asthmatic attacks. Glutaraldehyde can also exacerbate (aggravate) preexisting asthma and inflammatory or fibrotic pulmonary disease. Sensitized individuals may experience asthmatic responses following glutaraldehyde exposure to minute quantities of glutaraldehyde, well below the legal exposure limits.

Exposure in the dental office most commonly occurs during manual scrubbing of instruments, during retrieval of instruments soaking in precleaning solution, during mixing and preparation of the activated solution, from evaporation of the solution out of open containers into the ambient air, from application of solution to touch and splash surfaces such as countertops, from x-ray processing procedures, and during disposal down the sanitary sewer.

The National Institute for Occupational Safety and Health (NIOSH) has established a recommended exposure limit of 0.2 ppm, which should not be exceeded during any part of a work shift. Respiratory protection should be worn by all dental staff who may be exposed above this limit or during emergency work–related procedures.

Thus, the dental assistant is advised to use glutaraldehyde products carefully when proper controls are in place (Box 10-2) and

---

DID YOU KNOW?

Glutaraldehyde fumes are highly toxic; thus the dental assistant should avoid contact with these solutions with exposed skin or eyes and must not inhale the vapors.

If the dental assistant must work with glutaraldehyde, the following steps should be taken for adequate protection:

- Use glutaraldehyde in a separately designated area that is properly ventilated. Ideally, a local exhaust system should be installed at the point of glutaraldehyde vapor release.
- Keep containers of glutaraldehyde covered when they are not in use.
- Wear eye protection such as goggles or a full-face shield as well as a protective laboratory coat or apron.
- Wear protective gloves made with polyethylene. (Latex and neoprene gloves do not provide adequate skin protection from glutaraldehyde.)
- Wear appropriate respiratory protection (mask) if exposed above the NIOSH-established recommended exposure limits of 0.2 ppm (0.8 mg/m^3) or during emergency procedures.

Box 10-2 Guidelines for Protection When Working with Glutaraldehyde

following adequate training and using proper protection.

Iodophors

Iodophors are intermediate-level disinfectants. The dental assistant must take care when handling and diluting the solutions to derive the correct concentration. As the name suggests, iodine is a main ingredient of an iodophor and thus may cause staining of light-colored chair covers, countertops, and other surfaces with repeated use.

A second disadvantage of iodophors is they have the potential to corrode some metals; they also have a short life span and must be changed as often as every three days. They are also irritating to the ungloved skin.

Iodophors may also be used for dental instrument processing, requiring from 5 to 25 minutes upon contact (for disinfection only).

Sodium Hypochlorite

Sodium hypochlorite is another intermediate-level disinfectant and is derived from common household bleach, which is usually supplied in a concentration of 5.25 percent.

For general-purpose disinfection the dental assistant may use a 1 : 10 dilution, adding one-quarter cup of bleach to one gallon of water. Because of rapid deterioration, sodium hypochlorite used as a disinfectant must be discarded at the end of the workday and a fresh solution made the next morning.

Sodium hypochlorite may be corrosive to some metals and is irritating to the skin and eyes. The dental assistant must take care not to contact sodium hypochlorite with clothing because it may cause moderate to severe bleaching and in some cases may eat through clothing.

As when mixing, handling, using, or storing other chemical disinfectants, the dental assistant must take care to wear proper PPE and to avoid inhaling the toxic fumes.

Phenolics

Phenolics are also used for intermediate-level chemical disinfection. An advantage of phenolics is that the surface contact time is generally only 10 minutes.

Disadvantages of phenolics are that they are irritating to the eyes and skin and are destructive to plastic surfaces.

Isopropyl Alcohol

Also called isopropanol, **isopropyl alcohol** was once used as a surface disinfectant because of its low cost and quick surface drying time.

A disadvantage of isopropyl alcohol is that it has only limited disinfection properties; because it has a fast drying time, it does not provide sufficient time to be efficacious in many applications. Isopropyl alcohol is no longer recommended for disinfection in the dental office.

■ GASES: NITROUS OXIDE, OXYGEN, AND ETHYLENE OXIDE

While **nitrous oxide** (Figure 10-1), oxygen, and ethylene oxide may seem to be relatively harmless substances, they are inherently dangerous if not monitored or handled properly (Box 10-3). For women of childbearing years, miscarriage is the most commonly cited side effect associated with nitrous oxide vapors leaking into operatory air. Tanks must be stored away from heat and flame and in well-ventilated areas.

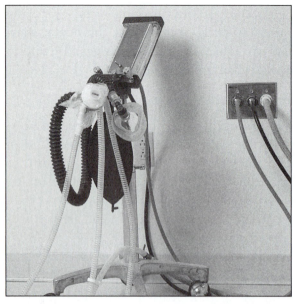

Figure 10-1 Portable nitrous oxide/oxygen unit.

The dental assistant must be vigilant at all times when nitrous oxide or oxygen is being delivered to a patient as well as when ethylene oxide gas is being used for instrument and equipment disinfection and sterilization.

Adverse Effects of Nitrous Oxide

Adverse effects associated with occupational nitrous oxide exposure in dental personnel have been well documented. Members of the dental team who routinely work with nitrous oxide are exposed to a two- to three-fold greater concentration of nitrous oxide than hospital personnel. Chronic exposure to nitrous oxide may result in nausea, perspiration, and hallucinations. Other documented adverse effects of chronic nitrous oxide exposure include reproductive problems, such as reduced fertility, spontaneous abortion, testicular changes, and decreased sperm count; neurological defects; hematological and immunological problems; liver problems; kidney problems; and cancer.

The dental assistant should follow these guidelines to reduce occupational exposure during conscious sedation administration:

1. Monitor anesthetic equipment when it is installed and every three months thereafter:
   - Test equipment for leaks.
   - Monitor air in the dental employees' personal breathing zones.
   - Monitor the environment (treatment room air).
2. Prevent leakage from the delivery system with proper maintenance and inspection of equipment. Eliminate or replace the following:
   - Loose-fitting connections
   - Loosely assembled or deformed slip joints and threaded connections
   - Defective or worn seals, gaskets, breathing bags, and hoses
3. Control waste nitrous oxide with a well-designed scavenging system that includes the following:
   - Securely fitting masks (Masks are available for your smallest to largest patients and their respective noses.)
   - Sufficient flow rates (45 liters per minute) for the exhaust system
   - Properly vented vacuum pumps
4. Ensure that the treatment room ventilation effectively removes waste nitrous oxide. If concentrations of nitrous are above 25 ppm:
   - Increase the airflow into the treatment room.
   - Use supplemental local ventilation to capture nitrous oxide at the source.
   - Institute an education program that describes nitrous oxide hazards and defines prevention measures.
5. Minimize patient conversation during use of nitrous oxide.
6. Use dental dam, where applicable, for procedures involving administration of nitrous oxide.

Box 10-3 Guidelines to Reduce Occupational Exposure During Administration of Nitrous Oxide

Methods to Reduce Occupational Health Hazards Associated with Nitrous Oxide

NIOSH recommends that dental practices control nitrous oxide exposure by inspecting and maintaining the delivery system to prevent leaks in hoses, connections, and fittings. All necessary repairs should be made immediately.

Dental practices should also use a scavenging system to maintain ventilation of the gas from the patient's mask at an airflow rate of 45 liters per minute, measured by a calibrated flow device. The system should be vented outside, not into the treatment room ventilation system.

Scavenging masks should be of proper size to fit patients. Nitrous oxide should be used prudently when providing patients with conscious sedation. The dental assistant should monitor the air concentration of nitrous oxide to ensure the controls are effective in achieving low levels during dental procedures (Box 10-4).

Guidelines for Safe Use of Oxygen

The dental assistant or safety supervisor should check the oxygen tanks weekly for faulty regulators (which can fail) or for leaking tanks. Consequences of neglect to check oxygen tanks can be disastrous. Extra oxygen in the atmosphere may cause objects to burn or explode. (By itself, however, oxygen is not explosive.)

Every dental office or clinic should have a minimum of two Series E oxygen tanks, which can be held upright in a portable carriage and secured so they cannot fall. The oxygen used in the office in conjunction with nitrous oxide in each treatment room is insufficient to deliver emergency oxygen in the

The dental assistant should follow these safety guidelines for oxygen use:
- Never use combustibles or flammables in the presence of oxygen, including petroleum products and nail polish remover.
- Never smoke or light matches near a source of oxygen.
- Do not store oxygen in temperatures exceeding 120°F.
- Never adjust the regulator with your body positioned directly over the tank.
- Connect the tubing to the tank and adjust the regulator before placing the delivery system (oxygen mask) on the patient's face.
- Do not deliver high concentrations of oxygen to those with chronic obstructive pulmonary disease because this may reduce their hypoxic drive.
- Post "Oxygen in Use" signs in treatment rooms where oxygen is routinely used.
- Avoid use of electrical appliances near oxygen because they may cause sparks, which can in turn cause an explosion.
- If oxygen tanks are used, they must be secured in a base or chained to a carrier or the wall.

Box 10-4 Safety Precautions When Using Oxygen

reception area, hallway, or elevator. Thus, a backup oxygen tank is essential because one tank may not last until emergency personnel arrive on the scene of an emergency.

How to Operate an Oxygen Tank

The dental assistant should follow these instructions regarding oxygen tank operation:
1. To turn on the tanks, attach oxygen delivery system to the tank.
2. Turn the key on the top of the tank in counterclockwise direction to open the flow of oxygen.
3. Read the low-flow regulator knob; turn in the direction the arrow indicates to increase or open. (Many regulators are

opposite of sink faucets and open clockwise instead of counterclockwise.)

4. Attach the oxygen delivery system to the person requiring it.

To turn off the oxygen, the dental assistant should do the following:

1. Remove the oxygen delivery system from the person using it.
2. Turn the key on the top of the tank in a clockwise direction to shut off the flow of oxygen.
3. Turn the low-flow regulator knob to the open position to bleed oxygen from the system.
4. After bleeding the system, gently close the low-flow regulator knob.

The dental assistant should always follow safety precautions when working with oxygen (Box 10-4).

Precautions for Using Ethylene Oxide

Ethylene oxide is a gaseous sterilant used in larger dental offices and clinics to disinfect and sterilize instruments and equipment. Ethylene oxide has been shown to cause mutations (changes), chromosomal aberrations (deviations from the norm), and fetal abnormalities. Ethylene oxide may also cause cancer.

Ethylene oxide is associated with an increase in spontaneous miscarriages and preterm and postterm births in female dental assistants with occupational exposure.

A dental office that uses ethylene oxide must provide adequate ventilation and proper protective equipment to staff who may contact this substance.

■ DARKROOM CHEMISTRY

An important role of the dental assistant is the exposure and processing of diagnostic-quality dental **radiographs** (also referred to as **x-rays**). (For additional information on the components of an x-ray machine, protection of operator and patient, and exposing and mounting of radiographs, refer to Chapter 17: Dental Radiography in *Delmar's Dental Assisting: A Comprehensive Approach,* second edition, by D. J. Phinney and J. H. Halstead, 2003, Clifton Park, NY: Thomson Delmar Learning.)

Developer and Fixer

The assistant must be familiar with the liquid radiographic processing chemicals, called **developer** and **fixer**. Whether using manual or automatic processing, the chemistry and outcome are similar (Figure 10-2).

Developer is a solution that removes the bromide from the metallic silver, which is chemically known as reduction. The black metallic silver that remains forms the image of the exposed object (teeth and supporting tissues).

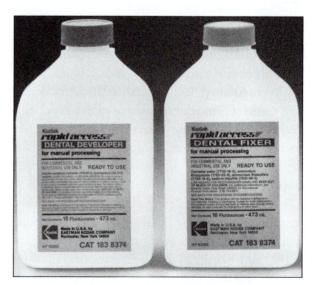

Figure 10-2 Bottles of manual processing developer and fixer solutions.

(Reprinted courtesy of Eastman Kodak Company.)

The purpose of developer is to bring out the latent (invisible) image of dental structures on an exposed (but unprocessed) film. Developer is comprised of hydroquinone, elon, sodium sulfate, and other chemicals.

After the exposed film is developed, it is rinsed in a water bath and is then fixed. During the fixing phase the undeveloped silver halide salts are removed by immersion of the radiograph in the fixer. The fixer is composed of sodium thiosulfate/ammonium thiosulfate, also referred to as hyposulfite of soda or simply as hypo.

Hypo acts as the fixing agent of the film. It removes the unexposed silver halide crystals that were not affected in the developing stage. Sodium sulfite acts as a preservative. Acetic acid compensates for the alkaline chemicals. Potassium alum is the hardening agent that reduces (shrinks) the gelatin that was softened and swollen during the developing phase (see Table 10-1).

Radiographic Processing Solutions

When mixing radiographic chemicals, the dental assistant should use distilled water (only) as other chemicals found in tap water have a potential to damage the silver halide (bromide) salts contained in the emulsion. When handling, mixing, or storing radiographic chemical solutions, the dental assistant should follow the manufacturer's directions.

Processing solutions are supplied in two differed forms: concentrated and ready to use. The dental assistant must dilute the concentrated chemicals with distilled water.

The ready-to-use radiographic chemicals are supplied in quarts and gallons. The ready-to-use chemicals are used in automatic processors. Either type of radiographic chemicals

should be stored in a cool, dark place, away from direct sunlight or heat.

Replacing and Replenishing Radiographic Processing Solutions

With regular use, radiographic solutions should be changed every three to four weeks. (Regular use is defined as 30 intraoral films per day.) Heavy workloads may require more frequent changes. The levels of solution should be checked and replenished daily, as necessary, to maintain solutions at the proper concentrations and levels.

In a practice that processes an average of 30 films per day, the following guidelines are recommended:

- For manual processing tanks (1 U.S. gallon/ 3.8-liter size) and for automatic roller-type processors containing 1 gallon (3.8 liters) of each solution, approximately 8 oz (236 mL) of replenishment is necessary daily for developer and fixer, each.
- Automatic roller-type processors with larger solution capacity require approximately 12 oz (355 mL) of replenishment daily.

If the practice or clinic processes more than 30 intraoral films per day, the dental assistant should increase the amount of daily replenisher solution at the rate of 0.25 oz (7 mL) per additional film processed.

Radiographic chemical solution life is based on three variables:

- Use factor—Greater use means shorter life.
- Exposure to air—Causes oxidation of the chemicals, which shortens effective life.
- Temperature—Chemicals deteriorate under extreme heat; they become inactive in extreme cold.

Thus, each variable—use, air, and temperature—deteriorates the activity of the radiographic solution. Fresh chemicals produce

Chemical	Action/Use	Purpose/ Characteristics
Developer		
Hydroquinone	Reducer	Slowly gains density by converting exposed silver halide (bromide) crystals to black metallic silver Highly sensitive to temperature changes
Elon	Reducer	Quickly brings the image to gain density Not highly sensitive to temperature changes
Sodium carbonate	Accelerator	Softens the gelatin of the emulsion Promotes developing Too little slows developing efficacy Too much may cause chemical fogging of films
Sodium sulfite	Preservative	Prevents oxidation Prolongs the life of the developer
Potassium bromide	Restrainer	Prevents too rapid development Prevents fogging of transparent areas on the film (due to unexposed silver halide crystals)
Fixer		
Sodium thiosulfate (hypo)	Fixing agent, clearing agent	Removes unexposed silver halide (bromide) crystals unaffected by the developer
Sodium sulfite	Preservative	Prevents deterioration of sodium thiosulfate
Acetic acid	Acidifier	Maintains acidity and neutralizes alkaline developer by stopping developer action
Potassium alum	Hardener	Hardens and shrinks gelatin

Table 10-1 Composition of Radiographic Developer and Fixer

better diagnostic-quality radiographs. Replenishing the solutions regularly over several weeks in small quantities helps maintain high-quality radiographs.

As an example, 50 intraoral films per day would require 13 oz (385 mL) to be added daily, that is, the usual 8 oz (236 mL) for the first 30 films plus an additional 5 oz (148 mL) for the additional 20 films.

Manufacturers of non–roller-type automatic processors recommend that all solutions be changed every two weeks.

Waste Management of Radiographic Chemicals

Most photographic film solutions, including developer and fixer, are biodegradable and therefore compatible with municipal waste–water treatment systems. Liquid waste radiographic chemistry should be carefully poured into a drain connected to a sanitary sewer system.

The dental assistant should take care to ensure compliance with applicable local waste regulations. Drains should be flushed or purged at the close of each clinical business day to reduce bacterial accumulation and growth.

Some practices contract with a licensed waste management company to pick up and dispose of used radiographic supplies.

■ HAZARD COMMUNICATION

Every dental office that has 11 or more employees is required by OSHA to have a written **hazard communication program**.

To comply with OSHA's Hazard Communication Standard, the dentist must develop and implement a written compliance program. This must include an exposure control plan (including the Bloodborne Pathogens Final Standard), a written hazard communication program, waste and sharps handling and management, and injury and illness prevention (Figure 10-3).

The dentist should designate a safety supervisor to provide staff training to new employees and once annually thereafter. The dentist must also maintain and update the written hazard communication program, develop ways to reduce hazards in the office, and provide a safe means for handling of hazardous materials.

Physical and Chemical Hazards in the Dental Office

Physical hazards are evident in dental equipment, open flames, radiation, ultrasonic devices, sterilization units, sharp instruments, and so on. Electricity is also a major source of physical hazard. All electrical equipment must be properly grounded, following the manufacturer's instructions and according to local electrical codes. All electrical cords and plugs must be kept in working order, with no frayed cords, exposed wires, or overloaded circuits. Extension cords should not be used except in an emergency.

Fire is another potential danger in the workplace, with fires occurring most often where open flames, such as Bunsen burners, are used. When using an open flame, such as for melting wax, the dental assistant must take care not to allow loose clothing or long hair to catch on fire. (For additional information on emergency fire evacuation and use of a fire extinguisher, refer to Chapter 15: Office Emergency Procedure in *Safety Standards and Infection Control for Dental Assistants* (by E. Dietz, 2002, Clifton Park, NY: Thomson Delmar Learning).

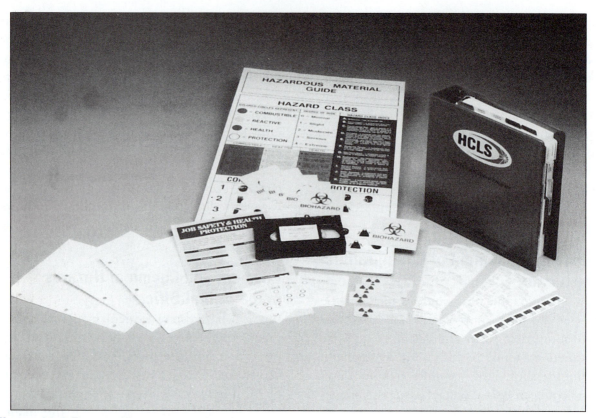

Figure 10-3 Every office must maintain an office manual with exposure control plans, training material, hazard communication, and OSHA-required employee records as part of a complete hazard communication program.

(Reprinted courtesy of Medical Arts Press.)

In other areas of the office hot plates, automatic coffeemakers, and microwave ovens should be used, rather than open flames. The dental assistant should store flammable chemicals in a flameproof cabinet away from heat sources and in a well-ventilated area.

The dental assistant must also take care when using pressurized sterilizers to prevent explosions and steam burns.

Material Safety Data Sheets

Chemicals present a variety of hazards in the dental office because they may be flammable, toxic, caustic, corrosive, carcinogenic, or mutagenic. The dental assistant or safety supervisor must make and maintain a hazardous chemical inventory of all products used in the office. These items must be appropriately labeled or tagged and have a corresponding MSDS on file that is accessible to all employees.

Manufacturers of chemicals are required by law to put hazard information on product labels and to provide corresponding MSDSs for every potentially hazardous chemical or material used in the dental office (Box 10-5).

Material Safety Data Sheets (Figure 10-4) describe the physical and chemical properties of a product, physical and health hazards, route of exposure, precautions for safe

OSHA requires each MSDS contain the following:
- Identification (chemical and common names)
- Hazardous ingredients
- Physical and chemical characteristics (boiling point, vapor pressure, etc.)
- Fire and explosion data
- Health hazard data
- Reactivity data
- Spill and disposal procedures
- Protection information
- Handling and storage precautions, including waste disposal
- Emergency and first-aid procedures
- Date of preparation of the MSDS
- Name and address of the manufacturer

Box 10-5 Material Safety Data Sheets

handling and use, emergency and first-aid procedures, and control measures. It is the dental office's responsibility to ensure that MSDSs are obtained on each hazardous substance used in the office, that they are kept up to date, and that all employees have access to them.

The dental office must also maintain a **hazardous materials log**, which is a list, a file folder, or a binder of all hazardous materials or substances used in the office as well as where each item is located in the office and the quantity on hand.

Product Warning Labels and Stickers

Hazardous chemicals used in the office must be properly labeled and other hazardous substances must have corresponding MSDSs. Under the revised hazard communication standard, all dental practices are required to communicate to their staff members the hazards of the chemicals they use in the practice. Labeling (Figure 10-5) is a key element of a sound and

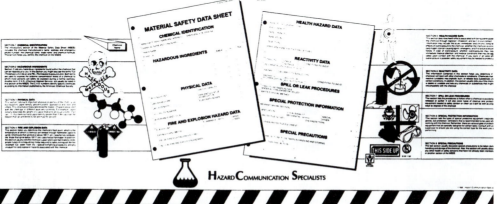

Figure 10-4 Material Safety Data Sheets (MSDSs) provide product information on hazardous substances used in the dental office. OSHA requires all dental staff to understand how to use MSDSs and where they are located in the office.

complete hazard communication program. Labels must provide a brief synopsis of the hazards of chemicals used in the practice.

Labels also help serve as a reminder to warn dental staff that the chemicals they contact require proper care, storage, and handling.

Chemical warning labels correspond to the information contained on MSDSs and identify the contents of containers of hazardous chemicals. They show hazard warnings appropriate for staff protection; for example, "Gloves must be worn when handling certain chemicals." All chemicals used in the dental office must be labeled. In the majority of applications, the manufacturer's label is

sufficient. However, if the chemical is transferred to a different container, a new label must be placed on that container if the material is not used up at the conclusion of an 8-hour work shift.

The label or sticker must contain appropriate warnings by hazard class, including routes of entry into the body and target organs of the body that may be affected. Product labels must contain the identity of the chemical, the appropriate hazard warnings, and the name and address of the manufacturer.

A container properly labeled when received from the manufacturer or supplier does not require an additional label. The exception for

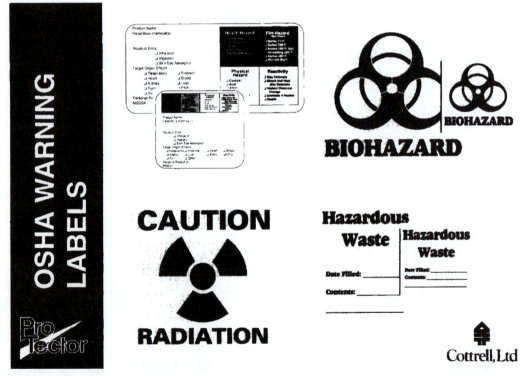

Figure 10-5 OSHA warning labels and stickers for hazardous products and devices and biohazard labels for hazardous waste.

(Reprinted courtesy of Cottrell Ltd.)

labeling is single-use or single-dispensing items or products.

All members of the dental team should familiarize themselves with the labels of hazardous substances and be aware of how to clean up spills or handle other emergencies that may arise when handling these products.

Fluorescent orange or red-orange **biohazard warning labels** contain the biohazard symbol. The word "biohazard" must be attached or affixed to containers of regulated waste and to refrigerators and freezers containing blood and other potentially infectious materials as well as to containers used to store, transport, or ship blood. Red bags or red containers may be substituted for labels as long as dental staff are trained to associate them with biohazardous contents.

Staff Training on Hazardous Chemicals

The dentist or owner of the practice is required to provide staff training regarding potential hazards inherent in the practice, including hazardous chemicals. This training must be provided for new employees at the beginning of employment, for employees of record whenever a new hazardous material is introduced into the office, and at least annually thereafter.

The dentist or owner of the practice is legally responsible to provide this training; however he or she may delegate training responsibilities to the office manager, the safety coordinator, or other team member.

Training must include the following:
- Hazards of chemicals and proper handling
- Operation where hazardous chemicals are used
- Availability of MSDSs

- Explanation of the labeling of hazardous chemicals
- Explanation of OSHA regulations

OSHA also requires that hazard communication training include methods and observations that may be employed to detect the presence or release of a hazardous substance in the work area (for example, continuous radiation, nitrous oxide monitoring devices, or particular odors associated with chemicals).

Physical and health hazards of these chemicals used in the work area must be addressed (for example, avoidance of handling mercury with ungloved hands or the potential for acid etch to burn skin or clothing).

Training must also include measures employees can take to protect themselves from hazardous materials using PPE, which must be supplied by the dentist or employer in appropriate sizes for all clinical staff members.

The dentist is responsible for explaining the details of the hazard communication program, including the labeling system, the use and nature of MSDSs, and how employees can obtain and use the appropriate hazard information for their safety.

Employee training may be conducted at staff meetings using audiovisuals, lectures, and videotapes or at continuing education courses offered through accredited providers. Training should be conducted in such a way that employees understand the information presented and that their questions are answered; training must be conducted at no cost to employees during standard working hours.

Hazardous Chemical Training Recordkeeping

Verification for training must be documented, indicating when and where the training took place and those present. Training records should be maintained for a minimum of three years and records must be available to employees upon request for review and copying (Box 10-6).

In the event the practice is sold or transferred, employee records must be transferred to the new owner. If the practice is permanently closed due to death or retirement of the dentist, these records should be offered (in writing) to NIOSH 90 days prior to the anticipated close of the office.

Reducing Hazards in the Dental Office

All members of the dental team are responsible for reducing hazards and the potential for hazards. This can be done by the following:

- Keeping the number of hazardous materials to a minimum
- Reading all product labels and following directions for use
- Storing hazardous chemicals in their original containers
- Keeping containers tightly closed or covered when not in use
- Avoiding the combination of two or more known hazardous chemicals (for example, mixing household chlorine bleach with ammonia may cause an explosion; inhaling the fumes may be fatal)
- Wearing appropriate PPE when using hazardous chemicals or when there is potential for accidental exposure on contact with body fluids
- Washing and thoroughly drying hands before and after wearing gloves
- Keeping the office well ventilated and avoiding skin contact with known hazardous substances
- Keeping a functional fire extinguisher in the office
- Knowing proper clean-up procedures in

Date: To: From: Hours:

Title/Topic: _____

Training Summary: _____

_____

_____

Safety Coordinator/Trainer: _____

Staff Members Present   Job Title

_____

_____

_____

Box 10-6 Staff Training Record

the event of a chemical or hazardous chemical spill (Figure 10-6)

- Disposing of all hazardous chemicals and other substances in accordance with MSDS instructions or the product label

The Exposure Minimizing Form (Box 10-7) provides a guide to outline and define the primary tasks performed by each staff member who may, as part of the nature of the job, have potential or probable exposure to hazardous substances or other potentially infectious materials.

The Engineering Controls column should include those types of equipment or safety devices used in the office to help minimize risks to employees. These may include scrubbing instruments with an ultrasonic cleaner, placing plastic barriers on treatment room equipment, or installing a protective shield on the model trimmer.

The Work Practice column should include measures taken by staff to eliminate or reduce exposure. These might include the following: avoid touching contaminated instruments directly, avoid inhaling glutaraldehyde fumes, or avoid using a model trimmer without a shield and face mask.

The PPE used for these procedures should be listed for each task, for example, gloves, eyewear, mask, and gowns.

Handling Hazardous Materials

Because contact with hazardous materials is inevitable when working in the dental office, there are measures the dentist and dental assistant can take to protect themselves. The

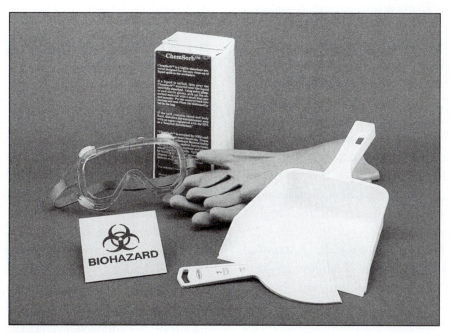

Figure 10-6 Emergency spill kit.
(Courtesy of SmartPractice, Phoenix, AZ.)

Each dental staff member who has the potential to contact hazardous chemicals or products should have an Exposure Minimizing Form on file. When the job duties or descriptions change, the form must be updated to reflect the changes or additions.

Name: _____ Job: _____ Date: _____

Tasks Assigned	Engineering Controls	Work Practice Controls	PPE Used

Box 10-7 Exposure Minimizing Form

most significant measure is using PPE, which is part of the universal precautions mandated by OSHA.

As part of the hazard communication program, the office must have a written procedure for handling and disposing of used or outdated materials that cannot be poured down the sanitary sewer or treated as routine or medical waste. These materials include but are not limited to outdated x-ray solutions, vapor sterilization fluid, lead foil from dental x-ray packets, scrap amalgam, and glutaraldehyde solution with a concentration higher than 2 percent.

Dental team members must be instructed how to handle spills and clean-up of hazardous substances and chemicals. In the event of an accidental spill, staff should follow the manufacturer's instructions (found on the label or on the MSDS) and wear appropriate PPE.

■ CRITICAL THINKING QUESTIONS

1. Why should the dental assistant wear protective gloves made with polyethylene when working with glutaraldehyde?
2. While nitrous oxide, oxygen, and ethylene oxide seem to be relatively harmless substances, when can they become inherently dangerous?
3. What are some of the reported dangers associated with occupational exposure to nitrous oxide?
4. What are the three variables upon which radiographic chemical solution life is based? Discuss each.

CHAPTER 10: POSTTEST

Instructions: For each of the following, select the answer that most accurately completes the question or statement.

1. Disinfectants used in the dental office may be harmful if inhaled excessively or used in areas with inadequate ventilation.
   A. True
   B. False

2. Which of the following is not a reason why contact of skin and clothing with disinfectant should be avoided?
   A. stinging or burning of the eyes
   B. stinging or burning of the skin or lungs
   C. pneumonia
   D. permanent discoloration of clothing

3. Which of the following should the dental assistant not do when handling sterilants and disinfectants (because of their toxicity)?
   A. follow the manufacturer's instructions for storing, diluting, handling, and disposal
   B. avoid wearing PPE
   C. follow instructions for proper shelf life and use life and dispose of all solutions according to local statutes and government requirements
   D. keep necessary clean-up and spill-kit materials handy in the event of an accidental spill or splashing of solutions

4. Which of the following statements is not true regarding chlorine dioxide compounds?
   A. They are EPA-registered, high-level chemical disinfectants and sterilants.
   B. They are EPA-registered, low-level chemical disinfectants and sterilants.
   C. Because of their corrosive property, chlorine dioxide disinfectants should be stored only in plastic or glass containers.
   D. When used as an instrument sterilant, 6–10 hours is required.
   E. They can only be used on instruments, environmental surfaces, and equipment not susceptible to corrosion.

5. Glutaraldehydes can cause mucous membrane irritation and asthmatic attacks as well as aggravate preexisting asthma and inflammatory or fibrotic pulmonary disease.
   A. True
   B. False

6. Latex and neoprene gloves provide adequate (skin) protection from glutaraldehyde.
   A. True
   B. False

7. Which of the following statements are true with regard to iodophors?
   A. are intermediate-level disinfectants
   B. may cause staining of light-colored chair covers, countertops, and other surfaces with repeated use
   C. have the potential to corrode some metals
   D. have a long life span
   E. may also be used for dental instrument processing, requiring from 5 to 25 minutes upon contact

8. Sodium hypochlorite is another intermediate-level disinfectant and is derived from common household bleach, which is usually supplied in a concentration of
   A. 1.25%
   B. 2.25%
   C. 5.25%
   D. 10.25%

9. When used as a disinfectant, sodium hypochlorite must be discarded at the end of the workday and a fresh solution made the next morning.
   A. True
   B. False

10. For women of childbearing years, _____ is the most commonly cited side effect associated with nitrous oxide vapors leaking into operatory air.
    A. acne
    B. miscarriage
    C. appendicitis
    D. hemorrhage
    E. asthma

11. Which of the following health problems is not a result of chronic occupational exposure to nitrous oxide?
    A. nausea, perspiration, and hallucinations
    B. reproductive problems, such as reduced fertility, spontaneous abortion, testicular changes, and decreased sperm count
    C. neurological defects
    D. hematological and immunological problems
    E. asthma

12. NIOSH recommends dental practices use a scavenging system to maintain ventilation of the gas from the patient's mask at an air flow rate of _____ liters per minute, measured by a calibrated flow device. The system should be vented outside, not into the treatment room ventilation system.
    A. 25
    B. 35
    C. 45
    D. 65

13. Patients with chronic obstructive pulmonary disease should receive higher concentrations of oxygen to help facilitate breathing during dental procedures.
    A. True
    B. False

14. The purpose of x-ray fixer is to bring out the latent (invisible) image of dental structures on an exposed (but unprocessed) film.
    A. True
    B. False

15. Which of the following is not a purpose or characteristic of sodium carbonate, a component of developer solution?
    A. It prevents oxidation.
    B. It softens the gelatin of the emulsion.
    C. Too much may cause chemical fogging of films.
    D. Too little slows developing efficacy.

16. To comply with OSHA's Hazard Communication Standard, the dentist develops and implements a written compliance program, including which of the following measures?
    A. an exposure-control plan (including the Bloodborne Pathogens Final Standard)
    B. a written hazard communication program
    C. waste and sharps handling and management
    D. injury and illness prevention methods
    E. all of the above

17. Manufacturers of chemicals are required by law to put hazard information on product labels and to provide corresponding MSDSs for every potentially hazardous chemical or material used in the dental office.
    A. True
    B. False

18. OSHA requires each MSDS contain which of the following information?
    A. hazardous ingredients and health hazard data
    B. physical and chemical characteristics (boiling point, vapor pressure, etc.)
    C. doctor's employer identification number
    D. spill and disposal procedures and name and address of manufacturer
    E. all of the above

19. Chemical warning labels correspond to the information contained on MSDSs and identify the contents of containers of hazardous chemicals and show hazard warnings that are appropriate for staff protection.
    A. True
    B. False

20. Staff training on hazardous chemicals must include which of the following?
    A. hazards of chemicals and proper handling
    B. operation where hazardous chemicals are used
    C. availability of MSDSs
    D. explanation of the labeling of hazardous chemicals and explanations of OSHA regulations
    E. all of the above

Dental assistant certification may be earned in one of several areas. Upon successful completion of the requirements set forth by the Dental Assisting National Board, Inc. (DANB), the dental assistant, office manager, or chairside assistant may use the credential Certified Dental Assistant (CDA) following his or her name and may wear the DANB pin.

DANB has established respective designations of certification, which include Certified Dental Assistant, Certified Orthodontic Assistant, Certified Oral and Maxillofacial Surgery Assistant, and Certified Dental Practice Management Administrator. Certification may be earned through a variety of eligibility pathways established by DANB for each. Regardless of the pathway selected or the type of certification sought, each pathway requires proof of current cardiopulmonary resuscitation (CPR) certification from either the American Heart Association or the American Red Cross.

To assist faculty and students, DANB periodically publishes an updated *Task Analysis* booklet (available for a minimal fee) to facilitate dental assisting programs in developing and designing curricula and learning experiences to prepare students to sit for one or all of the national certification examinations for dental assistants. Instructors and students should be aware that the items in the *Task Analysis* are periodically reviewed, revised, and updated as deemed necessary by DANB; test bank questions are reviewed and updated annually by members of the Test Construction Committee.

The General Chairside Certification Examination may be taken by individuals without prerequisites and DANB does not set eligibility requirements for it, although the *Task Analysis* provides competency prerequisites. Students should be aware that some states may require various eligibility standards because successful completion of these tests may complete that state's requirements for certification. The information contained in this text addresses only certain portions of the General Chairside Certification Examination and all requirements relevant to dental materials are addressed in this text.

Neither the author nor Thomson Delmar Learning holds responsibilities for content or changes in the DANB *Task Analysis.* Test applicants and program instructors are encouraged to periodically contact DANB to request updates. All attempts were made as of the publication date of this text to include interpretation of the latest requirements.

Note: Completion of the content herein does not imply a guarantee of successful completion or a passing score on any of the DANB certification examinations. Additional information about certification testing requirements, locations, and dates may be obtained by contacting the Dental Assisting National Board, Inc., in Chicago, at (800) 367-3262. On-line testing is available in some states. For additional information, visit the website at www.danb.org.

■ REFERENCES

Dental Assisting National Board (Spring 2001).
  Certified Press, 1(35).

TEXTBOOK FIGURES FOUND ON ACCOMPANYING STUDYWARE™ CD-ROM

The following figures from the textbook are provided on the StudyWARE CD-ROM in full color. These figures have been provided so that students can better see the consistency and texture of some of the materials that they will be working with and also see more clearly certain steps that are part of the procedures that they will be performing. Instructors may also find this feature to be useful, particularly if they wish to display the color photos onto a screen in the classroom.

Following is a list of the figures that are located in full color on the StudyWARE CD-ROM:

■ CHAPTER 1

Figure 1-2: Amalgam restoration

■ CHAPTER 3

Figure 3-1: Zinc phosphate powder and liquid dispensed onto a glass slab

Figure 3-6: Dental assistant holding the cement spatula blade against the glass slab

Figure 3-7: One-inch snap test

Figure 3-8: Zinc phosphate of puttylike consistency for use as a thermal base

Figure 3-9: Intermediate ZOE supplied in powder and liquid or capsule form

Figure 3-13: RelyX Unicem self-adhesive universal resin cement

■ CHAPTER 4

Figure 4-2: Predispensed, disposable amalgam capsules

Figure 4-3: Amalgam bonding kit

Figure 4-7: Discarding of excess amalgam

■ CHAPTER 5

Figure 5-4: Mixing alginate in a flexible bowl, spatulating out air bubbles

Figure 5-5: Loading alginate into a mandibular tray

Figure 5-7A: Loading the maxillary tray in overlapping technique to prevent air bubbles

Figure 5-7B: Smoothing alginate using wet gloved fingers

Figure 5-7C: Removing a small amount of alginate from the hard-palate portion of the tray

Figure 5-7D: Inserting the tray into the patient's oral cavity

■ CHAPTER 6

■ CHAPTER 7

■ CHAPTER 8

■ CHAPTER 9

abrasive material that cuts or grinds the surface leaving grooves and a rough surface, in the form of either powder or paste

abutment an anchor tooth, root, or implant used for the retention of a fixed or removable prosthesis; the teeth adjacent to a pontic in a bridge

accelerator a substance that begins a process or reaction; also refers to an impression material mixed with a base

acid etch technique a phosphoric acid solution is applied to a tooth (to alter the surface of the enamel by creating microscopic undercuts between the enamel rods), which allows for adhesion of dental materials to the enamel by brush, spray, or cotton pledget; a resin restoration is then placed

acidity the level of acidity, compared to alkalinity, of a substance; on the pH scale 7 is considered neutral

activator a chemical, usually an amine compound, that causes initiator molecules to become active and to begin a polymerization reaction

adhesion the force or attraction that holds unlike substances together through physical or chemical means

adhesive a material used to improve retention between two objects or substances; also known as a bonding agent

alkalinity having a pH of more that 7

alloy a combination of two or more metals

amalgam a permanent metallic restoration placed in posterior teeth, due to its ability to withstand chewing compression

amalgamation the chemical reaction that occurs between the alloy and the mercury to form the silver amalgam used for a posterior dental restoration

amalgamator a machine that mixes (triturates and mulls) dental amalgam and other dental materials used to restore teeth

armamentarium the equipment and supplies required to perform a procedure

articulate to match the maxillary to the mandibular occlusion together

articulator a mechanical hinge and frame that holds models of the patient's teeth to maintain the occlusion, representing his or her jaws; replicates the temporomandibular joints to which upper and lower casts of the dental arches may be attached to simulate oral functions

base material applied in a putty or thick layer between the tooth and the restoration to protect the pulp from chemical, electrical, mechanical, or thermal irritation; also one portion of an impression material mixed with a catalyst

baseplate a preformed semirigid acyclic resin material that temporarily represents the denture base

basic set-up the initial instruments required for all dental procedures: mouth mirror, dental explorer, cotton pliers, and periodontal probe; the latter is optional

biohazard warning labels contain the biohazard symbol, which must be attached or affixed to containers of regulated waste and to refrigerators and freezers containing blood and other potentially infectious materials (PIMs) as well as to other containers used to store, transport, or ship blood or other PIMs

bite registration an occlusal record of the relationship between the upper and lower teeth

bite registration (impression) wax used to record the patient's centric occlusion

bite rim several layers of baseplate wax attached to the baseplate to represent the space provided by teeth in normal occlusion, registering the vertical dimension for the denture and establishing the occlusal relationship of the mandibular and maxillary arches

biting force any push or pull on an object; the result is resistance. The reaction of the object to resist the external force is stress. When too much stress is placed on an object, this object is forced to change; this change is known as strain.

bonding agent a low-viscosity resin used to improve retention between two objects [in dentistry, between the tooth structure (enamel and dentin) and the restoration], also known as an adhesive or a bonding resin; usually light or auto cured

border molding when making a final impression, the impression compound is heated and applied along the borders of the patient's custom tray; the tray is cooled and inserted into the mouth; the patient's lips, cheeks, and tongue are moved to establish an accurate representation of the periphery and adjacent tissues to be replicated in the final impression

calcination the process of removing water from hard stone to create gypsum materials

calcium hydroxide a low-density cavity liner used as a direct or indirect pulp cap and to stimulate the growth of secondary dentin

carbamide peroxide a bleaching agent used to whiten teeth

cavity liner a low-strength base applied in the deepest portion of a cavity preparation on the dentin or exposed pulp that hardens to form a cement layer to protect the pulp from chemical irritation and to provide a therapeutic effect on the tooth

cavity varnish used to seal the dentin tubules to prevent acids, saliva, and debris from reaching the pulp; when used in conjunction with a cavity liner or medication, the cavity varnish is applied on top of these materials

cement base high-strength base of thick, puttylike consistency applied to the floor of the cavity preparation to protect the pulp and to provide mechanical support for the restoration; preparation, pulp sensitivity, and the type of restoration placed indicate the cement to be used

chlorine dioxide compounds EPA-registered, high-level chemical disinfectants (and sterilants) that can be used only on instruments, environmental surfaces, and equipment not susceptible to corrosion

composite a tooth-colored, direct restorative material used for both anterior and posterior teeth; it does not require the use of mercury

corrosion occurs as the result of chemical or electrochemical influences of the oral environment on metals, such as amalgam or gold

custom tray made from a variety of materials and can be fabricated using self- or light-curing acrylic resin, vacuum resin, or a thermoplastic material; fashioned from a stone model of the patient's mouth

denture base sometimes referred to as a saddle, denture teeth are held here

developer liquid chemical used to develop radiographs

die stone used in the dental laboratory for fabrication of crowns and bridges

dimensional change in a dental material occurs for a variety of reasons, including setting process, exposure to heat or cold associated with storage prior to activation, or exposure to foods or drink introduced into the oral cavity

direct pulp capping (DPC) a technique used to treat permanent teeth when the pulp has been exposed due to mechanical or traumatic means but the possibility exists the pulp will heal by itself; involves placement of medicament directly over the exposed pulp followed by restoration of the tooth

ductility the ability of a material to withstand permanent forces of tensile stress without breaking down or fracturing

elasticity the ability of a material to be distorted or deformed by applied force or the addition of a catalyst to that material; the material then returns to its original shape when the force has been removed

endodontic sealers and cements materials used to perform endodontic (root canal therapy) procedures

esthetics a pleasant or attractive appearance; an esthetic dental material is one that matches the patient's original dentition

ethylene oxide a gaseous sterilant used in larger dental offices and clinics to disinfect and sterilize instruments and equipment; it is known to cause mutations and cancer

exothermic reaction a chemical reaction in which heat is released

fixed appliance an appliance attached to the teeth than cannot be removed by the patient

fixer liquid chemical used to fix an image on a radiograph after developing is complete

flash extraneous material

flow sometimes referred to as creep, is a continuing deformation of a solid when it is under constant force

fluoridation the process of adding fluoride to the public water supply

fluoride a natural mineral proven to make the teeth more resistant to the caries process

4-META 4-methacryloyloxyethy trimellitate anhydride

full-cast crown full restorative covering over a tooth that has extensive decay, damage, or breakage

galvanism creation of electrical shock caused by two different metals through a conductor; for example, saliva is a conductor that creates a shock when gold and silver amalgam are used as restorations in the patient's mouth; this is referred to as a galvanic shock

gel the semisolid state of a hydrocolloid

glass ionomer cement a new cementation system, with a variety of applications in dentistry; supplied as powder and liquid, paste systems, syringes, and capsules; glass ionomers are also supplied in either self-curing or light-curing systems

glutaraldehyde a solution used for high-level disinfection and cold sterilization

gypsum rock-derived product delivered in a fine powder; used for a variety of dental laboratory procedures, including replicating oral structures

hardness the ability of a dental material to withstand or resist scratching or indentation

hazard communication program a written program that details methods used to reduce the incidence and minimize hazards that may be occupationally present in the dental office

hazardous materials log a file folder or a binder of all hazardous materials or substances used in the office as well as where each item is located in the office and the quantity on hand

HEMA 2-hydroxyethyl methacrylate

hydrocolloid impression material used for taking preliminary impressions of the oral structures; may be either irreversible or reversible

imbibition enlargement due to the absorption of fluid; a swelling

impression (bite registration) wax used to record the patient's centric occlusion

indirect pulp cap a soothing, medicated liner placed in the cavity preparation of a tooth that does not have a pulpal exposure

infection control methods and protocols used to eliminate or reduce the likelihood of transmission of infectious microorganisms

initiator a substance that contains molecules that cause or initiate a polymerization reaction

iodophors intermediate-level disinfectants

irreversible hydrocolloid commonly called alginate, a material made from seaweed used to make primary dental impressions

isopropyl alcohol (isopropanol) once used as a surface disinfectant

light cured process by which a resin or bonding agent is solidified

liner a material placed in a thin layer on the walls and floor of a cavity preparation

lute/luting to cement; the process of attaching one structure to another using an intermediate agent, such as cement or wax

malleability the ability of a metal being compressed to withstand permanent deformity without rupturing

Material Safety Data Sheets (MSDSs) written information about the content and potential hazard of specific products used in the dental office; each product in the dental office that has a potential hazard must have a corresponding MSDS on file in the office

matrix a mold or shape used in dentistry to replicate a natural tooth or teeth

mechanical retention the attachment of materials to surfaces by grooves placed in the cavity preparation by the dentist

mercury a metal that is liquid at root temperature; used to make an amalgam restoration

mercury vapor undetectable mercury molecules that may be released into the air; potentially hazardous and may be absorbed through the skin or through inhalation

microleakage occurs when saliva and debris from the oral cavity collect between the tooth structure and the restoration, eventually causing recurrent caries; it is the primary reason dental restorations must be removed and replaced

nitrous oxide a form of conscious sedation commonly used in the dental office to help patients relax; it is often used in combination with local anesthesia

NPE nonylphenol ethoxylate

onlay a restoration that overlays the cusps of the tooth

pathogenic disease causing

pattern wax sometimes referred to as inlay wax, used on a die, which is a positive replica of a prepared tooth poured in laboratory (die) stone

periodontal surgical dressing a material placed over the site of the surgical wound to act as a bandage while during the healing process; there are three types of periodontal dressings: zinc oxide eugenol, noneugenol, and light cured

personal protective equipment (PPE) items required for dental chairside personnel to wear during all invasive procedures; minimal standards include the donning of gloves, face mask, eyewear with protective side shields/goggles, and outer protective clothing, such as scrubs or laboratory coat

phenolics used for intermediate-level chemical disinfection

plaster (Plaster of Paris) one of the oldest (and weakest) gypsum products used in dentistry

polishing the process of using fine abrasives to produce a smooth, glossy surface

polycarboxylate cement (zinc polyacrylate cement) permanent cement used for crowns, bridges, inlays, onlays, and orthodontic bands and brackets

polyether impression material used in prosthetics

polymer a self-curing acrylic tray resin (powder)

polymerization the process by which a material changes from a plastic pliable state into a rigid state

polysiloxane/polyvinyl a dental impression material used when sharp detail is required; most often used in crown and bridge cases and for the fabrication of dental implant prostheses

polysulfide/rubber base a material used to make final impressions; comprised of a base and lead peroxide accelerator

pontic portion of a bridge that replaces the missing tooth or teeth

porcelain-fused-to-metal crown a crown that has a porcelain veneer for esthetics

processing waxes those most commonly used in dentistry include boxing wax, utility wax, and sticky wax

prophylaxis the procedure by which soft and hard deposits are removed from the teeth; this includes scaling and polishing

provisional restoration "serving for the time being" in anticipation of a permanent prosthesis; a temporary crown, either single unit or multiple unit

putty wash a technique in which a putty tray and impression material are used together as a final impression

radiograph a (dental) x-ray

radiolucent a dark area on a dental radiograph indicating where radiation has passed through the tissue

radiopaque a white or light area on a radiograph indicating where radiation was blocked by tissue or a substance

reline resurfacing of the underside or tissue surface of a full or partial denture to improve adhesion

removable appliance a device that is inserted and removed by the patient

resin cement a permanent cement used for cast crowns, bridges, inlays, onlays, and endodontic posts

retarder an added ingredient that slows setting time of the material

retention the process by which certain materials attach to hard and soft tissues in the mouth; retention may be either mechanical or chemical or both

reversible hydrocolloid used to make secondary dental impressions

sealant, pit and fissure a resin material mechanically bonded to pits and fissure of teeth to prevent caries

sedative palliative effect a soothing effect

self-curing a material that sets without the use of a specialty light by a chemical reaction

shelf life the amount of time a dental material is usable; prior to the expiration date marked on the packaging or label

silicone a final (secondary) impression material

sodium hypochlorite an intermediate-level disinfectant derived from common household bleach; it is usually supplied in a concentration of 5.25 percent

sodium perborate a bleaching agent used to whiten teeth

sol a liquid

solubility the ability of a substance to dissolve quickly or easily

spacer material placed on the teeth of a dentulous model or on the ridge and/or palate of an edentulous model to provide room for the impression material or tooth bleaching solution or gel

splint a custom appliance used to retain a traumatized tooth or teeth in position; also a tray used to deliver tooth bleaching liquid or gel to the teeth

stainless steel crown used in the restoration of a badly decayed or traumatized tooth; may be used as a temporary or permanent crown

stress the reaction of an object to resist an external force

(study) model a replica of the patient's oral structures poured in gypsum (stone) for use in prosthetics or orthodontics

study wax hard wax manufactured in blocks; used primarily for educational purposes to teach carving of teeth and dental anatomy

syneresis shrinkage due to a loss of water content from heat, dryness, or exposure to air

tactile pertaining to the use of touch

thermal conductivity the characteristic that determines the rate at which heat flows through a material; heat capacity is the amount of heat required to raise the temperature of an object by a certain amount

thermal properties characteristics of dental materials relevant to conductivity and expansion

thermoplastic reaction occurs when a material becomes pliable and soft when exposed to heat

tooth bleaching (whitening) a form of cosmetic dentistry, performed either in office or at home by the patient under the supervision of the dentist

toxicity (toxic effect) having a harmful effect upon a living tissue

trituration mechanically combining materials to form a dental amalgam restoration

triturator a mechanical device used to mix dental restorative materials, such as amalgam and certain types of composite; also referred to as an amalgamator

undercut a recessed area that is wider on the bottom than on the top

undercut wax used to fill undercuts of dental structures prior to taking impressions (to prevent the impression material from sticking to the prepared teeth)

universal (standard) precautions an OSHA standard requiring dental staff to treat all patients as potentially infected with a communicable disease and to wear personal protective equipment (PPE) when treating patients; minimal PPE includes gloves, a face mask, eyewear, and protective outer garments

vacuum-formed any appliance in dentistry that is fabricated using heat and a vacuum-former device; examples include secondary impression trays, athletic mouth guards, bleaching stents, and orthodontic appliances

varnish a thin layer of material placed to seal the walls and floor of a cavity preparation; some fluoride products are also available in varnish form

veneer a tooth-colored thin shell used to cover stained or misshaped teeth for esthetic appearance

viscosity the ability of a liquid to flow; the more viscous the substance, the stickier the substance, the less likely it is to flow quickly

wettability the capability of a material to flow over a hard or solid surface

zinc oxide eugenol (ZOE) cement a temporary cement or restorative material used for its palliative properties; sometimes used for full denture impressions

zinc phosphate a permanent cement used for crowns, inlays, onlays, bridges, and orthodontic bands and brackets

BIBLIOGRAPHY

American Dental Association (ADA) Council on Scientific Affairs and ADA Council on Dental Practice. (1996). Infection Control Recommendations for the dental office and the dental laboratory. *Journal of the American Dental Association, 127,* 672–680.

Anderson, P., & Pendleton, A. E. (2001). *The dental assistant* (7th ed.). Clifton Park, NY: Thomson Delmar Learning.

Dietz, E. (March, 2000). Is fungus lurking in the pumice? *The Explorer.* Falls Church, VA: National Association of Dental Assistants.

Dietz, E. (2002a). *Infection control techniques for today's dental assistant.* Falls Church, VA: National Association of Dental Assistants.

Dietz, E. (2002b). *Safety standards and infection control for dental assistants.* Clifton Park, NY: Thomson Delmar Learning.

Dietz, E.(2002c). *Mercury-amalgam safety and hygiene for the dental team member (continuing dental education course). Falls Church, VA: National Association of Dental Assistants.*

Dietz, E. (2003). *Provisional restorations.* Continuing education course prepared for GSC Home Study Courses, Sacramento, CA.

Dietz, E. (April, 2004). Fluoride varnish in six simple steps. *The Explorer.* Falls Church, VA: National Association of Dental Assistants.

Eastman Kodak Company. (1994a). *Exposure and processing for dental radiography.* Kodak Dental Radiography Series. Publication N-413. Rochester, NY: Eastman Kodak Company, Dental Products, Health Sciences Division.

Eastman Kodak Company. (1994b). *Waste management guidelines.* Kodak Dental Radiography Series, Publication N-417. Rochester, NY: Eastman Kodak Company, Dental Products, Health Sciences Division.

Ferracane, J. L. (2001). *Materials in dentistry: principles and applications* (2nd ed.). Baltimore, MD: Lippincott Williams & Williams.

Gladwin, M., & Bagby, M. (2000). *Clinical aspects of dental materials.* Baltimore, MD: Lippincott Williams & Wilkins.

Miller, C. H., & Palenik, C. (1998). *Infection control and management of hazardous materials for the dental team* (2nd ed.). St. Louis, MO: Mosby.

Phillips, R. W., Moore, K. B., & Swartz, M. (1994). *Elements of dental materials for dental hygienists and dental assistants.* (5th ed.). Philadelphia, PA: W. B. Saunders.

Phinney, D. J., & Halstead, J. H. (2001). *Delmar's handbook of essential skills and procedures for chairside dental assistants.* Clifton Park, NY: Thomson Delmar Learning.

Phinney, D. J., & Halstead, J. H. (2003). *Delmar's dental assisting: A comprehensive approach* (2nd ed.). Clifton Park, NY: Thomson Delmar Learning.

Williams, H. (February, 1997). A fungus lurks among us. *Lab Management Today,* pp. 737–739.

Intraoral radiography. *See* Darkroom chemicals
Inventory control, 18–19
Iodine-containing disinfectant, 17, 18, 233
Iodophors, 17, 18, 129, 130, 233
Irreversible hydrocolloid dental impressions. *See* Hydrocolloid dental impressions, irreversible
Isopropanol, 233
Isopropyl alcohol, 233

J

Journal of the American Dental Association (JADA), 2

L

Labels, warning, 241–243
Laboratory. *See also specific materials*
  commercial, 15–17
  dental laboratory prescription, 15–16
  dental materials in, 2
  disinfection of, 17–18
  office-based, 14–15, 16
  PPE in, 15
Latex examination gloves, 10, 11, 122
Laundering reusable protective garments, by employer, 13–14
Light, translucency of dental materials, 5–6
Light-curing techniques
  acrylic resin trays, 180–181
  ambient light effects, 48
  calcium hydroxide cavity liner, 27
  composite restoration, 87–89, 91
  dental cements, 48
  eyewear, 88
  periodontal surgical dressing material, 213
  resin cements, 32, 33
  sealants, pit and fissure, 206
  silicone impression materials, 123
Liquids. *See* Mixing and manipulation
Log, commercial laboratory cases, 15–16
Lost-wax technique, 170
Low-copper alloys, 80, 81
Luting, 48

M

Macrofill (fine) composites, 88, 89
Maintenance of dental materials, 3
Malleability of dental materials, 6
Manipulation. *See* Mixing and manipulation
Manufacturers of dental materials. *See specific dental materials*
Masks, 9, 10, 12, 13, 234–235
Material Safety Data Sheet (MSDS), 87, 240–242, 243, 245, 246
Matrix, 190
Measuring devises, for material manipulation. *See* Mixing and manipulation
Mechanical retention, 8
Mercaptan, 117
Mercury restorations, 85–87

vs. composite restoration, 88
defined, 85
dental alloys, 80, 81
mercury hygiene practices, 86–87
safe handling guidelines, 86
spill clean-up guidelines, 87
toxicity, 9
Metals as dental materials, 3, 4, 6, 7, 80, 81
Microfill composites, 88, 89
Microleakage, 7–8, 30
Miscarriage, and dental gases, 233, 234, 236
Mixing and manipulation
  acid etching, 37
  alginate impressions, 107–109, 110–111
  amalgam restorations, 82–85
  bonding agents, 37
  calcium hydroxide, 28
  calcium hydroxide cavity liner, 28, 29
  cavity varnish, 31
  composite restorations, 88–89, 90–91
  condensation silicone elastomeric impressions, 122–123, 124–126
  glass ionomer restorations, 60–62, 93
  hydrocolloid impressions, irreversible, 107–109, 110–111
  hydrocolloid impressions, reversible, 116
  of ideal dental materials, 3
  periodontal surgical dressing material, 213–214
  polycarboxylate cements, 57–59
  polyether impressions, 127–129
  polysiloxane and polyvinylsiloxanes elastomeric impressions, 122–123, 124–126
  polysulfide elastomeric impressions, 117–120
  provisional acrylic custom restorations, 190
  resin cement, 33
  sealants, pit and fissure, 206–207
  silicone elastomeric impressions, 122–123, 124–126
  thermoplastic acrylic resin trays, 182–184
  tooth bleaching, 212
  zinc oxide eugenol (ZOE) cements, 53–54, 57
  zinc phosphate cements, 52
Models. *See also* Dental resins
  custom resin tray fabrication, 180
  diagnostic cast, trimming, 106, 151, 154–158
  pouring alginate impression, 150–154
  type II, laboratory or model plaster, 148, 149
MSDS (Material Safety Data Sheet), 87, 240–242, 243, 245, 246
Mycobacterial germicide, 14–15, 17

N

Nanotechnology, 88
National Institute for Occupational Safety and Health (NIOSH), 232, 235, 244
NIOSH (National Institute for Occupational Safety and Health), 232, 235, 244

Nitrile utility gloves, 11
Nitrous oxide, 233–235
Noneugenol periodontal dressing, 213, 214–215
Nonsterile (disposable) examination gloves, 10, 11
Nonvital "walking bleach technique" bleaching, office-based, 209, 210–211

O

Odor free, dental materials as, 3
OPIMS (other potentially infectious materials), 10
Oral cavity, ideal materials for, 2–3, 4–9
Ordering inventory, 18–19
Orthodontic stone, 149
OSHA Occupational Safety and Health Administration, 9, 13, 239, 240, 241, 242, 243
Other potentially infectious materials (OPIMS), 10
Outer garments, disposable protective, 13–17
Outgoing laboratory cases, managing, 16
Overgloves, 10–11
Oxygen, 233–234, 235–236

P

Paper, large sheets of, for infection control, 17
Paper pad, for material manipulation. *See* Mixing and manipulation
Paper pad mixing. *See specific dental materials*
Passive vital tooth bleaching, home-based, 209–210, 212–213
Pastes. *See* Mixing and manipulation
Pattern waxes, 170
PEMA (polyethyl methacrylate), 189
Periodontal surgical dressing material, 213–216
  composition, 213
  mixing/manipulation, 213–214
  practice assessment and posttest, 227–228
  practice procedure: noneugenol dressing application, 214–215, 225–226
  properties, 213
  uses of, 213
Personal protective equipment (PPE), 9–15, 246
Phenolics, 17, 18, 233
PH of oral cavity, and dental materials, 4
Phosphoric acid, 4, 9, 34–35
Photocured system. *See* Light-curing techniques
Physical adhesion, 3, 4, 30. *See also* Bonding agents
Physical hazards in dental office, 239–240
Pit sealant. *See* Sealant for pits and fissures
Plaster of Paris, 148–149
PMMA (polymethyl methacrylate), 189
Polycarboxylate cement, 57–59
  composition, 57
  defined, 57
  mixing/manipulation, 57–59

Minimum System Requirements:

- Operating System: Microsoft Windows 98 SE, Windows 2000 or Windows XP
- Processor: Pentium PC 500 MHz or higher (750Mhz recommended)
- RAM: 64 MB of RAM (128 MB recommended)
- Screen Resolution: 800 x 600 pixels
- Color Depth: 16-bit color (thousands of colors)
- Macromedia Flash Player V7.x.
  The Macromedia Flash Player is free, and can be downloaded from http://www.macromedia.com

Installation Instructions:

1.   Insert disc into CD-ROM player. The *Materials and Procedures for Today's Dental Assistant StudyWARE™* installation program should start up automatically. If it does not, go to step 2.
2.   From My Computer, double click the icon for the CD drive.
3.   Double-click the setup.exe file to start the program.

Technical Support:
Telephone: 1-800-477-3692, 8:30 A.M.-5:30 P.M. Eastern Time
Fax: 1-518-881-1247
E-mail: delmarhelp@thomson.com

StudyWARE™ is a trademark used herein under license.